NEW
Atomic Power With God
Thru Fasting and Prayer

(Enlarged and Revised Edition)

BY FRANKLIN HALL

author of

OUR DIVINE HEALING OBLIGATION

THE FASTING PRAYER

BECAUSE OF YOUR UNBELIEF

For price list and address of author—see back page

PRAYER AND FASTING IS JESUS CHRIST'S MESSAGE
TO HIS PEOPLE EVERYWHERE

A STUDY OF THE SCIENCE OF FASTING
IN RELATION TO THE GREAT SPIRITUAL
PHYSICAL AND SPIRITUAL POWER OBTAINED THEREBY

INTERDENOMINATIONAL   NON-SECTARIAN

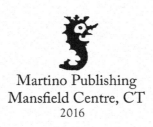

Martino Publishing
Mansfield Centre, CT
2016

Martino Publishing
P.O. Box 373,
Mansfield Centre, CT 06250 USA

ISBN   978-1-61427-946-4

© 2016 Martino Publishing

Cover Design Tiziana Matarazzo

Printed in the United States of America On 100% Acid-Free Paper

NEW

Atomic Power With God

Thru Fasting and Prayer

(Enlarged and Revised Edition)

BY FRANKLIN HALL

author of

OUR DIVINE HEALING OBLIGATION

THE FASTING PRAYER

BECAUSE OF YOUR UNBELIEF

For price list and address of author—see back page

PRAYER AND FASTING IS JESUS CHRIST'S MESSAGE TO HIS PEOPLE EVERYWHERE

A STUDY OF THE SCIENCE OF FASTING
IN RELATION TO THE GREAT SPIRITUAL
PHYSICAL AND SPIRITUAL POWER OBTAINED THEREBY

INTERDENOMINATIONAL   NON-SECTARIAN

WORLD-WIDE REVIVAL
THRU PRAYER AND FASTING
By FRANKLIN HALL

Historic developments are underway in the body of Christ. The Holy Spirit is pouring out His gifts in an unusual way. In recent months we have been privileged to see mass salvation-healing meetings where nearly everyone prayed for, was delivered. Not only hundreds but sometimes thousands of unbelievers find Christ in a single revival campaign.

Surely there must be a cause behind the present spiritual awakening. Where there is even a spiritual condition, there must be a cause. Has Christendom made strides in any direction, it has not made in past years? Why have not we had these greater experiences years ago? These and other questions might be asked, yet there is a very definite answer that will explain the great manifestation of the Spirit, that we are witnessing now.

There is a spiritual law that is applicable to God. We have noticed that He never moves, without His creation moves first. If they move in a wrong direction, then man must suffer the consequences as in the judgments that fell on Sodom and Gomorrah, and the flood that came upon the people in Noah's time. We have a contrast to this, with the city of Nineveh. Judgment was already pronounced by God. It would be overthrown in forty days, but the whole city repented and sought God, by proclaiming a fast. The city was spared. God reversed His decision.

God's people, for the last number of years were in an almost powerless condition. There were few mighty revivals and but little power and demonstration of His Spirit. Denominational walls were created and prejudice existed everywhere.

Every spiritual person knew something was wrong, but what was the lack? Many were praying dead prayers. Faith was dead and without works.

In the very beginning of 1946 a group of Holy Ghost people from many different denominations met together in all night prayer meetings and started fasting and praying longer than at any other time since the time of Christ. Some fasted ten, twenty-one and forty days. Some went longer. They were burdened for an old time world-wide revival of power, and the gifts of the Spirit—gifts of healings, where diseases would vanish and demons would be cast out, etc. Fasting and prayer was taught and it spread everywhere, beginning in Southern California. Many books and tracts were printed. There was a great demand to know more about it. Then Fasting-Prayer revival crusades started. Soon thousands of people all over the world began fasting for the old time revival power of healings and signs following.

What could not be accomplished without Jesus Christ's truth of fasting and prayer was very definitely accomplished by the utilization of this vital process. A result is always traced to its cause. Many who were burdened and carried forward this fasting-travail, are now rejoicing, seeing the hand of God move forward. This resulted in moving much UNBELIEF FROM THE BODY OF CHRIST. Even those who did not have a special part in it are also reaping benefits today. These history making events were also prophesied in Joel's prophecy of which we are now living. (Joel 2 and 3).

Fasting and prayer by thousands of the Lord's people paved the way for the great SALVATION-HEALING CAMPAIGNS THAT FOLLOWED A YEAR LATER IN 1947, AND THE SPIRITUAL AWAKENING THAT IS BEING SEEN AMONG GOD'S PEOPLE EVERYWHERE. Preparation is being made for Jesus' soon return.

Much mis--understanding, confusion and abuse existed in people's minds in regard to the subject of fasting. More enlightenment was necessary so more Christians could understand about a subject that had been hidden in plain sight for more than 1900 years. Jesus graciously supplied the needs in order to put out four million pieces of literature and two hundred thousand books (up to the present time), which almost entirely dealt with this truth. Seldom anything was ever published before upon the subject. The first book written was, "ATOMIC POWER WITH GOD," in the early part of 1946. This was the year the fasting crusade began. It has since gone all over the world.

There is no time to let up. Still greater, yes much greater things than ever before are in the making, if men and women continue to fast, pray and get down to business with God. Veneering will not do. We must have reality in our fasting and prayer. We must converse with God. We should see even greater triumphs for our Lord, because we have no confidence in ourselves, but our confidence is in God. Our Jesus wants more daring men and women—those who will dare all and be strong in Him, to courageously step out and do exploits.

We wish to express our appreciation to members of the Lord's body everywhere for helping to do their part in spreading (world-wide) this glorious part of our Jesus' message, fasting and prayer.

JAMAICA

(As given to the author while visiting with Brother and Sister Osborn in their new house trailer during their wonderful tent cathedral campaign in Reading, Pa. where 3,000 souls found Jesus as their Saviour and many hundreds were healed from all manner of diseases.) The East was stirred by this campaign. Thousands packed around the tent.

*We are happy to let you know that we feel our lives have been revolutionized by fasting and praying to Jesus. It was through your books getting into our hands, that enabled us to go into many days and weeks of fasting and praying. Both my wife and I have had many deep fasting and prayer experiences. My life was changed so that God began using me in the healing ministry. As I began to exercise the ministry of praying for the sick, it seemed that more and more folk were healed.

One day while in deep consecration the Spirit spoke thus: "My son, as I was with Price, Wigglesworth and others, so will I be with thee. They are dead but now it is time for you to arise, to go and do likewise. You can cast out devils; YOU heal the sick; YOU raise the dead; YOU cleanse the lepers. Behold I give you power over all the power of the enemy. Be not afraid. Be strong. Be of good courage. I am with thee as I was with them. No evil power shall be able to stand before THEE all the days of thy life, as you get the people to believe my Word. I used those men in their day, Now I desire to use THEE."

The challenge of this commission given directly from the Lord caused me to tremble exceedingly, but I knew God meant every Word He had spoken.

More days and weeks of fasting and prayer followed this tremendous commission, and more healings and miracles were the result.

We have been able to conduct Healing Campaigns already in over a dozen of our states on the Island of Jamaica, B. W. I. In a single campaign which we conducted, as many as one hundred-twenty-five deaf-mutes, ninety totally blind and hundreds of other equally miraculous deliverances have resulted. Happy and joyful conversions have numbered as many as nine thousand in one revival.

We found people all over the island acquainted with your books and tracts. Many were fasting and praying for this revival before we came.

Brother Hall, we wanted you to know, we do appreciate your vision, and the

---

*(BROTHER OSBORN'S FIVE DIFFERENT BOOKLETS ON FAITH HEALING POWER CAN BE ORDERED FROM HIM AT THIS ADDRESS AT $.50 cents per copy. They are invaluable and many receive healing while reading. Write to him for literature.) T. L. OSBORN, BOX 4231, Tulsa 9, Oklahoma.

tremendous way you have STIRRED THE WORLD with FASTING AND PRAYER. We shall do all we can to push that part of the Gospel. We are going to handle your book in our meetings and shall order them in large quatities. You may send me one thousand of your, "Because of Your Unbelief," revival booklets.

We are planning on going into other countries with the message of deliverance, in the near future.

Yours in Christ for the DELIVERANCE OF ALL
T. L. OSBORN
Box 4231—Tulsa 9, Oklahoma

SOUTH AFRICA
From Missionary Department

June 11, 1948
Administrative offices
7 De Villiers Street
Johannesburg, South Africa

Beloved Brother in Christ:

Your books have been a real blessing and inspiration to my soul and many are already testifying of great blessings that they received through the reading and practicing of the protracted fasts. God has graciously helped me to complete a 24-day fast with much blessing and a new revelation for His work.

The message God has given you in your books has come in these closing days of time to do a great work for Him. I want to encourage you to go on with the job.

My Mission called for a Mission-wide fast for 21 days, and on one Sunday during that time about 60,000 people were fasting and praying. Many went the full length and fasted for 21 days and even longer.

We have testimonies of wonderful healings. One young man was released from a Leper Institute, perfectly healed. Another child who was paralyzed received healing and can now walk. Another was healed of the T.B. of the bone, another of stomach cancer; another who was involved in a motor accident and was unconscious for 18 days was healed and is now one hundred percent well. There are other outstanding healings coming in daily, that are too numerous to mention.

We have noticed reports from all over this continent how a revival tidal wave is coming about through fasting and prayer. We give Christ the glory.

With Warmest Christian Greetings,
Yours in His Royal Service,
F. J. Hawley
MISSIONARY SUPERINTENDENT

AUSTRALIA-NEW ZEALAND and AFRICA

Dear Brother Hall: July 1, 1948

Greetings to you in the Name of the Lord!

As you will see by this letterhead, I am the Australian Secretary of the Russian and Eastern European Mission, and by the magazine forwarded under separate cover, the Editor of an Australian magazine called, "THE EVIDENCE." Mr. Chas. R. Bilby is manager of our New Zealand Office and they have been in touch with you in connection with your books.

At present I am visiting South Africa, although at the moment I am writing from Rhodesia, where I have three campaigns booked in the three largest towns of Salisbury, Bulawayo and Umtali.

Your books and literature on prayer and fasting have helped me a great deal.

Recently I had a 23-day fast as per the enclosed article. You are welcome to use this if you wish. (See August, 1949 issue of "The Voice of Healing" for an account.)

In addition to this fast the last eleven campaigns in South Africa and Rhodesia I have started with a call to the people to fast and pray. The response to this appeal has been most encouraging, and the mighty blessings experienced as a result of the fasting have been remarkable. Eight of these campaigns were started with a three day fast, and the other three with a two-day fast.

I would prefer a long fast instead of many short fasts, but as these campaigns are only for a week, I have felt I was accomplishing more by speaking to new people each week and getting them to fast with me. It has all been very wonderful. Three days fasting each week is about as much as one can manage.

Fasting in AFRICA has been given a great deal of emphasis in behalf of an international revival. *Brother Hawley,* the missionary Superintendent of the Apostolic Faith Mission, from whom you have received letters and who has distributed a great number of your books, has done a great deal in this respect.

He recently had a 24-day fast. A letter from his assistant yesterday, Brother Eric Wilson, tells me of another 20-day fast that he has just completed, which is his second long fast this year. Recently there was an urgent call sent out by Brother Hawley right through the Union of South Africa for a time of fasting and prayer, to which approximately 60,000 people responded.

God bless you in the work you are doing. You have indeed been the instrument in God's hands to awaken many thousands in many countries to this wonderful truth, that is so clear in the Word of God and yet so neglected.

With every kindest wish in the Lord,
Brother Len J. Jones, 197 President Ave.,
Kogarah, Sydney, N.S.W., Australia

UNITED STATES

*"We believe that there is a great truth in prayer and fasting, since Jesus, when speaking of the devil in the lunatic child whom the disciples could not heal, declared, 'this kind cometh not out but by prayer and fasting.' We do realize that fasting to be seen of men for self-aggrandizement is futile and profitless. But fasting with prayer has a place, as the Scriptures plainly teach. We know of no writer whom God has so signally used to bring out Scriptural truth on fasting, as Evangelist Franklin Hall. We feel that 'Atomic Power With God' is the book of the hour for believers. We trust that this book will be an especial help to those whose prayers, for one reason or another, have not been answered."

Brother Gordon Lindsay
Box 4097—Shreveport, La.

FASTED 40-DAYS AND RECEIVED GIFTS TO HEAL

Dear Brother in the Lord:

I am so happy for the Lord Jesus' truth of fasting and prayer.

After entering and completing a forty-day fast on March 30, God has helped in many miraculous ways. Since then Jesus has healed a regular landslide of CANCERS. One had cancer of the brain and two brain tumors. The work of Satan goes out quickly when prayer is made for these sick folk. The Lord is healing every kind of

---

*In recent months Brother Gordon Lindsay has been used with remarkable success in CITY-COMMUNITY-WIDE EVANGELISTIC HEALING CAMPAIGNS in auditoriums and tent cathedrals all over the country. His splendid, undenominational paper, "THE VOICE OF HEALING", can be had for $1.00 a year. Box 4097—Shreveport, La.

disease imaginable after the fast. I surely do recommend fasting to every minister who wishes to have a more successful healing ministry.

After just breaking another short fast of seven days, the Lord's power is all around the place where our prayer band meets.

I am director of "GOD'S WORLD PRAYER BAND" having approximately two thousand members. I would like very much to get your tracts on fasting and prayer into their hands. Will you please send me a quantity?

(Editor's note: It is prayer-fasting groups like these that are doing more than eye can see to bring a world revival.)

Sister May Eversole sends in a report of more fastings

Dear Brother Hall:

O, yes, I put into practice my faith in God. We are on a small fast now. I believe in it. Jesus did not show us how to do something that will kill us. I get very much out of fasting.

You are doing a nice work and it is helping to bring a world-wide revival of heal-ings and signs and demonstration of God's Spirit.

Thanks for the tracts. I have such a wonderful testimony. One time after finishing a twenty-eight-day fast, the Lord performed a miracle. I had a lot of bills to meet with no money to pay them. The God that multiplied the loaves and fishes, multiplied real money in my pocket-book. I opened it and there was over $200.00 in it. I could pay my bills. Our prayer band is travailing, fasting and praying for a world revival.

> Humbly, your Sister in Christ,
> Sister May Eversole,
> Director of "God's World Prayer Band"
> 1705 So. Cheyenne
> Tulsa 14, Oklahoma

CANADA—NEWFOUNDLAND

"It is with great interest and a very special delight to give my whole-hearted recommendation to this completely NEW and DIFFERENT BOOK on the most important and ALSO MOST NEGLECTED SUBJECT IN THE REALM OF CHRISTIAN LIVING, 'FASTING AND PRAYER.'

Certainly, our author has had a very definite calling of God and unusual insight into the most desired prayer of every earnest Christian—obtaining answers to prayer, and 'POWER WITH GOD.'

After reading the 'first sheets' before publication, in my own experience, IT HAS BEEN WORTH MORE THAN ITS WEIGHT IN GOLD, and I'm positive that every earnest reader will acquire new and priceless knowledge on the most valuable information on how to secure a position with God SO THAT FAITH WILL 'MOVE THE MOUNTAINS' in your life.

The blessed contents of this book are by far the most complete and easily understood of all knowledge upon this subject that I have read in all other books combined.

I count it a privilege indeed to have found such 'inspired treasures' to give the true light on 'FASTING AND PRAYER.' THE 'SPIRITUAL VITAMINS' in this MASTERPIECE will bring forth 'SPIRITUAL GIANTS' and overcomers for God and 'The Latter Rain will be here as at Pentecost.' "

One year later: After having fasted forty days and my wife, Barbara, twenty-one days, we have a far greater ministry in the Lord. Especially is this true concerning divine healing.

We have seen auditoriums packed out in Canada and Newfoundland. Hundreds were converted and healed from all kind of diseases. Many have fasted previous to these great meetings — for days and weeks at a time. We feel that a world-wide move is on.

> Your Servant in Christ,
> Evangelist, Dale Edward Hanson
> P.O. Box 795 Tacoma, Wash.

TABLE OF CONTENTS

CHAPTERS

CHARTS

Note: All Charts Drawn and Designed By Franklin Hall

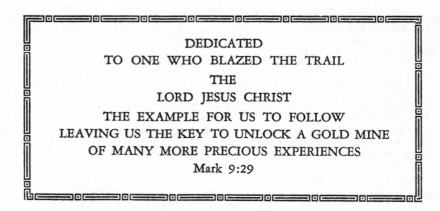

DEDICATED

TO ONE WHO BLAZED THE TRAIL

THE

LORD JESUS CHRIST

THE EXAMPLE FOR US TO FOLLOW

LEAVING US THE KEY TO UNLOCK A GOLD MINE

OF MANY MORE PRECIOUS EXPERIENCES

Mark 9:29

Chapter I

ATOMIC POWER WITH GOD

Fear and hatred stalk the world today, because no one knows to what use men will put the newly discovered force of atomic energy. Many other devices of power would bring to pass the signs preceding the second coming of Christ as foretold in Luke 21:26: "Men's hearts failing them for fear for the powers of heaven shall be shaken." Back of it all is the sad, irrelevant fact that man's spiritual development has lagged far behind his scientific discoveries of the physical forces of nature.

Spiritually and emotionally, mankind on the whole is not far removed from the jungles, and therefore, incapable of handling the forces of nature that science has unleashed. Physical power, sufficient to disintegrate the entire world, is at the fingertips of a few, but there has been almost no development of spiritual power to control it. We have been wandering in the wilderness.

This spiritual power is actually in the reach of all followers of Christ. It is not so much forgotten, but rather it has never been taught and learned. "The Gospel, and the message of the Gospel is the power of God unto Salvation." Rom. 1:16. But we have overlooked a certain fundamental of the Gospel.

The writer shall endeavor to present a power far greater than the physical force of all the atoms in the universe. Jesus Christ has made this power available to all His people, who will follow His Gospel pattern.

In 1848 A.D. the Aquarian Age was introduced to the world. The era of invention began and the machine came into being, along with the age of SPEED. Space and time began to shrink with the modern automobile, steam engine, and airplane. Distance ceased to be a barrier. More progress was made in two generations than had been accomplished in the preceding two thousand years of scientific achievement.

What about spiritual power? Outside of a sprinkling here and there of the Holy Spirit, and of power, scientific achievement has far out-distanced man's gains in things of the Spirit.

Surely if man's scientific achievement has increased in momentum, there must also be something somewhere in the Word of God to accelerate his SPIRITUAL PROGRESS. Like most scriptural truths, there is something; but only the wise shall understand it. The seemingly insignificance and misunderstanding may have been cause for its neglect. This latent power is FAST-ING AND PRAYER. This is a prayer that is prayed under the influence of fasting.

In the natural we have the automobile to speed us on our way. We have the steam engine shortening distance and also the airplane making distance no longer a barrier, etc.

Thank God there is something which makes for Spiritual progress that is more scientific than anything man has accomplished to date, and which ac-

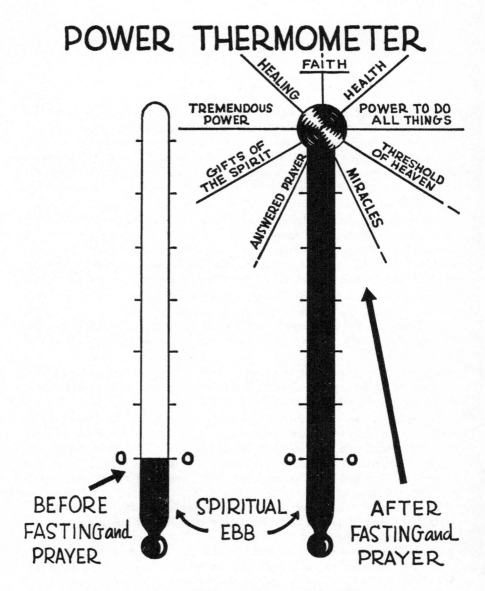

POWER THERMOMETER

FAITH

HEALING   HEALTH

TREMENDOUS POWER   POWER TO DO ALL THINGS

GIFTS OF THE SPIRIT   THRESHOLD OF HEAVEN

ANSWERED PRAYER   MIRACLES

BEFORE FASTING and PRAYER

SPIRITUAL EBB

AFTER FASTING and PRAYER

CHART No. 1. THE POWER THERMOMETER

THE LEFT SIDE OF THE CHART DOES NOT MEAN THAT ALL CHRISTIANS ARE COMPLETELY POWERLESS BEFORE UNDERTAKING A PROTRACTED FAST. THE CHART SIMPLY REVEALS THE AVERAGE STATE OF AFFAIRS WHICH THE ORDINARY CHILD OF GOD IS IN BEFORE FASTING. The Holy Spirit is useless to us if we fail to pray, or fast and pray. Divisions also enter the Body of Christ (Rom. 16:17, 18). Fasting and prayer brings unity and fills us with the glory of God.

8

complishes more for our Spiritual welfare in a short time. Without this knowledge this goal might not be attained for many years or perhaps NEVER. That something is FASTING AND PRAYER. A prayer intensified by fasting.

Our ultimate aim and desire should be in EXALTING JESUS CHRIST and GLORIFYING HIM. Without doing this every Christian will more or less fail in their purposes. The most successful method is through PRAYER AND FASTING; this pleases Jesus and in pleasing HIM we are availing ourselves of GREAT OPPORTUNITIES. "Delight thyself in the Lord; and He shall give thee the desires of thine heart." Ps. 37:4.

FASTING AND PRAYER will make it far easier to DELIGHT OURSELVES IN THE LORD, it will give us the light ON THIS POWER. SPACE AND TIME TO GOD WILL SHRINK AND DISTANCE WILL CEASE TO BE, when one receives the potential light and puts it into practice.

If the unleashing of atomic energy is the prelude to the end of the earth (as is mentioned in Luke 21), and the seals, trumpets, and vial judgments of the Revelation of Jesus Christ, then the few who know and experience the saving power of God would do well to protect themselves against the day of His Coming by a last great awakening through fasting and prayer.

It can only be the beginning of a new age for good if the power of the Spirit is developed to a high degree in many by the most powerful agent known to man, FASTING AND PRAYER. Without fasting, prayer becomes inefficient. Fasting restores and amplifies prayer power. Psalm 35:13.

A twenty-one, or forty-day Prayer and Fast period will most assuredly hasten the Christian to such a great and deep experience with God that twenty-one days would be equal to twenty-one years. Forty days equal to forty years (Experience shows that the forty day period gives far greater results than a shorter time) as far as the power of God is concerned, "and this would very likely be minimized, because the power obtained thereby is like Atomic power," and will bring one closer to God more quickly than any other way known.

The practice of fasting is as old as humanity, but like the doctrine of divine healing, the doctrine of the Holy Spirit, etc., this has been sadly neglected. Many other forgotten Bible truths have been temporarily lost, only to be revived again in these "latter days" of this dispensation, the transition period between this and the millennial dispensation. The truth of fasting is being *revealed to us now to secure the greater things of God, such as the "Gifts of the Spirit"* and a mighty world-wide revival of spiritual power that is definitely coming, as well as major signs and miracles in these last days. Fasting is the most potent power of the universe placed at the disposal of all believers. A transformation in the body of Christ will begin as Christians fast and pray.

More than two thousand years ago, fasting was a custom advocated by the school of the natural philosopher, Asclepiades, for curative purposes. Even Plutarch said, "Instead of using medicine, fast a day." Traces of this idea are to be found in ancient Chinese and Hindu writings. The Indians practiced it also. It was used for religious purposes, as well as a method of restoring health.

In the olden days they recognized the value of a fast but today people look at fasting as a certain way to the grave. When a person speaks of fasting ten days, twenty-one days or more, as they used to do, many think it something horrible. It is a definite lack of knowledge on the part of many that this subject is misunderstood.

Fasting is a CORNERSTONE of the CHRISTIAN RELIGION, yet there is seldom, if ever, a complete sermon on the subject up to the present time. Moreover, it is an important, basic-truth of the Bible; yet we often overlook the value of the process.

So important is fasting in the Mohammedan religion that they claim it to be one of the four pillars of the Mohammedan faith. This explains one of the reasons why there is more fervor and zeal in their religion than that of the Catholic and Protestant religions. Many Mohammedans take a thirty day fast every year.

Fervor and zeal is definitely a result of the fast and is sadly lacking in the church today.

Fasting is mentioned in the scriptures approximately one third as much as prayer, yet its practice in comparison, is placed insignificantly in the background.

If Christians realized what great power and blessings they are missing, they would be only too eager and happy to fast. However, one of the reasons Satan cheats them out of this glorious experience, is because of the misunderstanding and confusion that is generally prevalent in regard to fasting.

Here is a testimony of a certain gentleman who fasted fourteen days in one of my meetings. (This was when the world-wide fasting crusade was first launched).

UNDERWEIGHT—GAINS 29 POUNDS AFTER FASTING

"On the thirty-first day of December, 1945, after hearing Rev. Franklin Hall give some enlightening teachings on fasting, I started a consecration fast. I partook of no food during the entire fast of fourteen days. Water was taken for the purpose of cleaning out the system. I was a heavy smoker and it seemed it was impossible to give it up, but on the third day of the fast I had no further desire for smoking. On the fourth day of the fast, hunger left me entirely. A little later all weakness; and to my surprise I began feeling better and stronger day by day. I could pray more earnestly and with greater results. Several days later I received the glorious baptism of the Holy Ghost. I kept busy with my work which was not heavy, but fasting did not bother me much. What Brother Hall tells you about fasting is true and it worked out just that way in my life. It was a glorious experience.

When I began the fast, I weighed one hundred forty pounds, this was twenty-nine pounds underweight. At the conclusion of the fast which was fourteen days later, I had lost sixteen pounds, for I weighed a hundred and twenty-six pounds. Sixty days later *I had not only regained the lost weight but also gained twenty-nine pounds more,* which was exactly what I was supposed to weigh to the pound, or one hundred sixty-nine pounds.

Every one told me that I looked better than they had ever seen me look, and I do feel better than I have felt for twenty years. All of my nervousness is

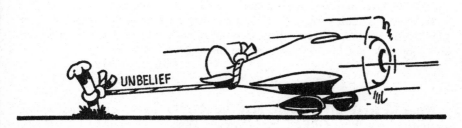

THE BONDAGE OF UNBELIEF

No. II. Showing that DOUBT, UNBELIEF, and the lack of FAITH prevents one from "taking off" and obtaining the greater things that God has for those who will ONLY BELIEVE. MANY CHRISTIANS ARE NOT GETTING THEIR PRAYERS ANSWERED, ARE NOT BEING HEALED IN ANSWER TO PRAYER, AND ARE NOT SEEING THEIR LOVED ONES SAVED, JUST BECAUSE THEY FAIL TO HAVE "THE FAITH" THAT IS BROUGHT ABOUT BY PRAYER AND FASTING. MANY PRAY, BUT HOW MANY WILL FOLLOW JESUS' COMPLETE FORMULA and FAST with their prayers, or go into THE FASTING PRAYER?

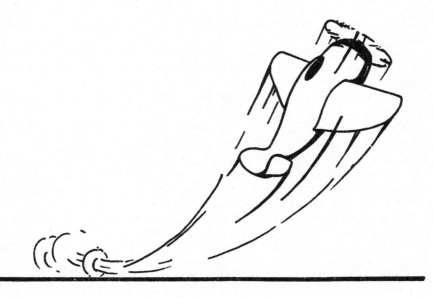

FAST AND TAKE OFF

No. III. This shows what will happen when the doubts and unbelief disappear through THE CONSECRATION FAST. The Christian gets "HIS SPIRITUAL WINGS." HIS UNANSWERED PRAYERS BECOME ANSWERED. DIVINE HEALING IS A DEFINITE FACT, ETC. JESUS IS EXALTED. One becomes a conductor of spiritual and supernatural power.

11

gone and I have better complexion, but the best part of all, I have received the Holy Ghost and have a much greater experience with the Lord.

My fast was shorter than many of the other brothers and sisters, but some day I hope to take a forty day fast, as it certainly was a glorious experience and people do not know what they are missing."

Charles Wilson
4010 Euclid Ave.
San Diego 5, California.

When we speak of "ATOMIC POWER WITH GOD" we are using a term expressing something GREAT, and "Atomic Power" is as good an expression as we could possibly find to fill the bill. We are not exaggerating in the least when we compare "FASTING AND PRAYING" with the power of the ATOMIC BOMB, because to the Christian this will bring even greater power. Atomic power is refractionated power. Fasting is likewise refractionated power from God.

ATOMIC BOMB

Robert deVore in Collier's, quotes some of the figures released by the mission of investigation in Japan on THE ATOMIC BOMB: (The Nagasaki and Hiroshima bombs probably detonated at about 1800 feet altitude)

"At 2,500 feet from point of impact— if bomb had reached earth—NOT from the point of explosion, 1,800 feet above, which would be farther—the pressure exerted was approximately SIX TONS TO THE SQUARE FOOT.

"At 4,200 feet, the pressure was a little more than ONE TON PER SQUARE FOOT.

"The first pressure noted above is equivalent to a gale force of wind of 150 miles per hour multiplied by 133—to the pressure of a wind blowing 20,000 miles per hour.

"The second pressure noted is equivalent to 24 times the pressure of a 150 mile gale (3,600 miles per hour).

"These enormous pressures are not wholly instantaneous, but are slightly delayed in their application, giving the water time to partially yield, and hence build up enormous wave effects. A vast, cone-shaped vortex will be created, with a terrific outthrust and subsequent return of the displaced waters. No one can possibly calculate the true extent of this effect, but some physicists have stated that a wave of great height will be created.

"Consider the effect on water of the temperatures developed. The temperature of the atomic "SUN" is estimated at FOUR MILLION DEGREES Fahrenheit. Materials of all kinds will (combustible) burn at 1.4 miles distance. The ground temperature below the burst (at 1800 feet altitude) was certainly more than 1500 degrees Centigrade. WATER WAS INSTANTLY CONSUMED," says DeVore. "Forests were scorched at 8,000 feet distance. All these facts point to the instant vaporization of MILLIONS OF TONS OF WATER, to be thrown far into the upper atmosphere, and thence reprecipitated in torrential falls in distant parts of the world."

"This isn't a bomb at all," says General Farrell.

"These are the Fires of the Universe," says physicist Walter Graham.

This is the GREAT NATURAL POWER MAN HAS DISCOVERED. THE

PURPOSE OF THIS VOLUME IS TO SHOW TO THE CHRISTIAN EVEN A GREATER POWER FOR HIS SPIRITUAL PROGRESS THAT CAN DEFINITELY BE OBTAINED THROUGH "FASTING AND PRAYER." This is a revival power that is within our very finger tips.

Chapter II

WHAT IS FASTING?

Let us see what the word FAST means: I believe herein lies much of our trouble about the subject of fasting, whereby Satan deceives the average individual.

Webster's and also the Bible Dictionary defines fasting as that of, "abstinence of food. Especially as a religious observance." (FAST: "To abstain from food"). Now what does Webster say about water pertaining to food, or we may ask the question, "Is water food?"

First we will consider Webster's definition of food, and it reads as follows: "Food: nutriment; nourishment in solid form." If you will notice the definition of nourishment, you will again find it to be food.

Food and drink are two different things. To do without water is thirsting, and thirsting means, "a great desire to drink." Fasting will be clarified if we recognize these facts. One should never associate abstinence from water with the subject of fasting; thus, we notice the contradistinction between food and water.

The confusion that exists in the mind of the Christian who believes that he is not to drink water in a fast, MUST be overcome. This has prevented many people from fasting over a period of several days. Therefore they have been deprived of some of the very greatest blessings to be had.

We will describe the protracted fast, or a "Complete Fast." We are dealing with the fast described and taken by the Lord Jesus Christ. A fast like that of Paul or Daniel; "A Bible Fast." A complete fast will be a fast from the time hunger leaves until the time when hunger returns. The fast might continue from twenty-one to forty days depending on the individual, and also on the amount of time it takes you to get your prayers through to Heaven.

Fasting and Starvation are also two entirely different things.

DRINK WATER WHEN FASTING

To take a fast of this particular type, one must of necessity drink water. It is absurd for people to think about fasting and prayer without drinking water. Those who do this, do it in ignorance, and should be corrected by some constructive teaching. However, one may attempt a fast of several days without drinking water and find these facts to be immaterial.

Your body is the temple of the Holy Spirit, and to attempt a major fast without water would defile and pollute the body. Scripture states: "If any man defile the temple of God, him shall God destroy." I Cor. 3:17.

Instructions are given by Christ in the Sermon on the Mount (Matt. 6:16-18) that "when thou fastest, anoint thine head, and *wash thy face;* that thou appear not unto men to fast, but unto thy Father, which is in secret, and thy Father which seeth in secret, *shall reward thee openly."* Washing the face is a sign of cleanliness. If it is good to wash your face to keep the toxic stains from face and body (washing being a type of cleanliness before God) then how much more logical it is to put water in your mouth to clean out the corruption in the stomach. The stomach becomes deflated, collapsed, and depressed when water is withheld long enough, and a person gets into bad shape. Without water, when fasting, the system will choke up, and the body becomes filthy.

The tongue, which is the upper part of the stomach, becomes heavily coated when fasting, showing a part of the pollution that is in the stomach. Some doctors maintain that some food particles remain in the intestinal tract for more than a month.

For the first few days of the fast, the stomach, tongue, and body, become heavily laden with the corruption that is trying to loosen itself. These particles that have remained in the stomach unassimilated, with other fecal matter, require a great deal of water to break them down and help soften this material so that it can be eliminated. Cramps, displeasure, misery and other discomforts are frequently experienced during this initial period.

Water aids in the loosening and softening up of this fecal matter without which the corruption will harden; the worms and bugs which are nearly always there to some extent will dry up on the intestines, the tongue will eventually thicken, and if the thirsting fast is prolonged, the individual will die, unless the Lord intervenes.

Paul knew the difference between "thirstings and fastings," he distinguishes their difference in II Cor. 11:27, "in hunger and thirst, IN FASTINGS OFTEN." If "hunger and thirst" were the same thing as "fasting," he would not have repeated the same thing, any more than "cold and nakedness" are the same. Please note that a "comma" is inserted after each description.

A person should not only recognize the value of the fast, but whether your fast continues ten days, two weeks, forty days, or longer, your bowels should move approximately every day or so. If a person does not drink water while the fast is in progress, how can these channels of elimination function properly? The drinking of water will continue the process of cleaning while the fast continues.

The drinking of water does not prevent one from drawing closer to God. Water is pure and is a type of Salvation and of the Holy Spirit. (Jno. 4:14). Water, unlike corruptible food, evaporates into the atmosphere, while food goes back to the earth.

Water is not stimulating, while food is. Food feeds the appetites of carnality, water does not.

When an individual fasts, his pores become laden with toxins, especially his hands and face, therefore, he should bathe externally as often as possible.

In about two weeks, more or less, the average individual will have most of the wastes, poisons, toxins, fecal materials, etc., eliminated. That is, unless this individual has a deep-seated functional ailment. Even if this be the case, this should be relieved if the fast is continued.

It is quite evident that Jesus took water while fasting forty days. There are four things that bear evidence in this regard. Shall we study our Lord's fast?

1. Matthew 4:2-11: "When he had fasted." We pointed out the *definition of fasting* that it did not exclude water drinking, and it does not mention that Jesus thirsted forty days in the scriptures, etc. It is called a fast and not a thirst.
2. "He was afterward an hungered." It does not say that He afterward thirsted. When a person does without both food and drink, water means far more to him than food. A man can go days without food, but this same individual can go but a very short time without water. Especially is this true in a hot and torrid clime.

   It seems very evident that Jesus did drink water. For at the time of the feeding the 4,000 (Mark 8:3), bread and fishes were offered after they had been fasting for three days, Jesus, according to all scriptural knowledge, never offered them water, because they had no need of water. Water was available in the springs and brooks nearby.
3. Satan knew that He wasn't thirsty, because he did not tempt Him with water. He said, "Command that these stones be made bread."
4. The answer that the Son of God gave to Satan, is very evident. "Man shall not live by bread alone, but by every word that proceedeth out of the mouth of God." This seemed to prove that He had partaken of water, for we must notice at this position the failure to mention water.

You may ask if the fast that Jesus took was a supernatural one, No, this fast was not in any form a supernatural fast, for fasting is not supernatural whether it is done by our Lord or by the ones He paid the great price to save. "FASTING IS A SCIENCE." Anyone can fast for long periods of time, but only the Christian can expect supernatural results.

The fast of Jesus can be said to be natural on the grounds that after His fast He hungered. The natural hunger that had left his body for a time returned again. This is true in any fast, if the fast be prolonged so as to allow this situation to start and complete itself.

Critics who say that only Jesus could fast forty days, while no one else could do so, are condemning something they know nothing about. They are in need of trying a fast themselves; then they would realize with a great awakening the value of fasting.

The argument is brought to us that Moses fasted forty days. Please tell me what scripture states this?

In Exodus 34:28-29, we read, "And *he was there with the Lord forty days and forty nights;* he did neither eat bread, nor drink water." This abstinence was not called FASTING HERE, as failing to drink water is outside the meaning of the word. Why change the meaning of the word FASTING?

On the mount, Moses was "there with the Lord for forty days"—this explains why Moses did not drink water—he was with the Lord, literally with the Lord.

I am certain that if we were allowed to stand in His presence and be with God, we would neither have to eat, drink, or breathe, whether we were with Him forty days, or forty years. Actually the Lord Himself is our Food, Drink and Sustainer.

This was true with Moses, because (Vs. 29)—"The skin of his face shone while he talked with Him." The children of Israel were actually afraid of Moses.

15

For he had received some supernatural radiation that was far more real than food and drink. He had to veil his face to talk to them. When Moses died, he had the strength and constitution of a young man.

If any person fasts without taking water, and he can do so if he wishes to, I must say, "Amen." However, any person can take short fasts of several days without water or food and still receive spiritual benefits for their sacrifice. See Esther 4:16.

Doing without food will give you that spiritual uplift and power, with or without water. This has been proven many times. This fact is true in the fast of a few days, but we are dealing with the long fast, which will give one power to do mighty things, seemingly the impossible, the fast that is "Atomic" Spiritual Power. The fast that will break down denominational barriers and restore the body of Christ to its place of power and unity of the faith.

Dr. Tanner, who fasted over forty days on three occasions, declared that in the second half of each of the three fasts, the unspeakable glories of the world beyond were revealed to him. Dr. Tanner lived to be ninety-two years of age, and gave credit to fasting for his longevity of life. In Dr. Tanner's day they ridiculed Christ's fast, saying "nobody could fast that long." Dr. Tanner challenged them. His first fast lasted over forty days and was under observation by his disbelievers. He was weighed and checked daily; thus he broke down the ridicule of fasting in his time. Dr. Tanner was a physician as well as a Christian. His first fast was so glorious that later on he took additional fasts of over forty days. After his last fast a crop of new black hair appeared in place of the grey hair.

Luther fasted for days at a time while translating the Bible, and herein undoubtedly lies the secret of his unrivaled translation and it is also responsible in bringing a reformation revival in his time. His great faith was likewise largely the revelation of God's presence, which comes only through PRAYER AND FASTING. Thank God for men that get a vision, who will press on all the way.

Chapter III

THE BACKGROUND FOR REVIVAL

"SANCTIFY A FAST, CALL A SOLEMN ASSEMBLY:" Joel 2:15

To see our loved ones saved, souls converted and a sweeping revival come in our midst, to have God work miracles and heal our diseases and the Holy Spirit poured out, we have to start a fast and prayer in the home. "LORD, let it begin in me!" Even if you are the only converted member of the family you can get a hold on God in such a way by FASTING AND PRAYING that Jesus, seeing your fervor and zeal developing the faith for your loved ones, will most certainly hear your prayer and convert them. Many times a person has done this and not only were the loved ones converted but the Lord so rewarded them that an "old fashioned" revival swept the whole community, saving, healing, and blessing mightily with the Holy Spirit.

In 1932 the Holy Spirit led the author into his first revival meeting. He knew only three families in the Oklahoma oil town, Nowata. One of these families believed and practiced FASTING AND PRAYER. Together we prayed and fasted ahead of time for the meeting that we knew God was going to give us there. The foundation was properly laid for a revival and a revival we certainly did have. There was no building big enough to take care of the crowd so we secured three acres of ground and had an open air meeting (this was in July). People packed the place from the first service. We kept building seats and the crowd continued to increase every evening. People gathered from all over Northeastern Oklahoma and Southeastern Kansas for the meetings. Scores of people were healed of all types of afflictions. One lady who had been in a car wreck with broken ribs was carried to the services on pillows; she was instantly healed. A deaf and dumb boy was instantly healed. A man who could not lift his arm and had been paralyzed was also healed; many more received notable healings. Folks were under the power of His Spirit. Many were baptized in the Holy Spirit.

Within three months from the time we started the meeting, we built a church and got it paid for so the people could continue to have a place to worship in truth and in Spirit. ALL OF THESE RESULTS WERE TRACED DIRECTLY TO PRAYER AND FASTING. My brother, Virgil Wm. Hall, assisted me in the meeting, and the church is still progressing for the glory of God to this day.

PASTOR FASTS TEN DAYS AND 300 CONVERTED

MEN ARE LEARNING HOW TO RECEIVE GIFTS

Dear Brother Hall: June 14, 1949

Some time ago a friend sent me one of your books, "Atomic Power With God." I was only a little interested when I first received it, but it grew on me. The anointing of God was upon your message.

Just recently I fasted into my tenth day, and along with my Bible I kept your book near. The Lord met me in a wonderful way during this fast; however I was forced to quit far too soon. My pastoral work took up too much of my time. When I fast again I expect to take it during my vacation, so that I can devote my full time to waiting on God.

The above book was studied during a recent fast by a friend of mine. In ONE WEEKS REVIVAL SINCE THESE FASTS, THREE HUNDRED PEOPLE WENT INTO OUR PRAYER ROOMS FOR SALVATION. I HAVE SEEN MORE OF GOD'S POWER MANIFESTED SINCE YOU HAVE WRITTEN YOUR BOOKS, AND MORE MEN LEARNING TO GET HOLD OF GOD FOR SPIRITUAL GIFTS THAN AT ANY OTHER PERIOD I KNOW SINCE THE TIME OF CHRIST.

Please send me your other books . . .

Yours very truly,
Pastor Harvey L. Smith
P.O. Box 262
Pascagoula, Mississippi

FASTING FOR THE HOME

If church leaders and parents, the heads of churches and homes, do not live up to "THE FAITH WHICH WAS ONCE DELIVERED UNTO THE SAINTS" (Jude 3), how do we expect our children to be saints? FASTING WAS AS SURELY A PART OF THE FAITH that was once delivered unto the saints as anything else. Fasting is one of the great foundation piers of the Christian religion. The structure of the Christian religion is built upon the vital truth of prayer and fasting. It was a vital part of the early church. Therefore, the great results that accompanied it were seen.

This explains the great "falling away," the "losing their first love," etc., because man, cares more for his "desire-nature" than for the fortification of his soul. People have failed to follow the complete pattern of the formula of Christ, Given in Matthew, chapter seventeen, or Mark 9:29, to have the "FAITH." They not only failed to have power to do the impossible, but the church, after the days of the apostles, became powerless, and eventually began to say that the days of healing were over; that the miracles were not for them anymore; the Holy Spirit, after the Bible pattern was forsaken with the power of the apostolic age. Many splits soon entered the church of Jesus Christ. The men of old that had fasted and prayed, and who had power with God to perform miracles and healing, had either died, or were martyred.

Matt. 9:15: "The days will come, when the Bridegroom shall be taken away from them, and then shall they fast." How many "Children of the Bridegroom" are obeying Christ's command, "then shall they fast?" This is where the Lord lays a fast upon us.

It wasn't as necessary to fast while Jesus was here on earth, because He had fasted to obtain the more perfect faith. After He left we could have had thru FASTING the same power and FAITH that His visible presence gave.

Many, if not all, the American Indian tribes sought revelation of the Great Spirit through Prayer and Fasting. When Indian tribes had famines, food shortages, and lack of rain, etc., the Great Spirit was sought in prayer and fasting, and their prayers were answered.

In certain tribes nearly all Indian children who came to the age of puberty, were required to be set aside in a prayer and fast of seven to ten days, to burn out, so to speak, the evil sex desires, so that they would have high moral thoughts, and live a high spiritual life. As they grew and developed into manhood or womanhood this practice was continued.

This should be a lesson for the American home today. If this method were taught and put into practice in our day, we would not see so many disobedient sons and daughters who are the source of such grief and heartaches to their parents.

A survey was recently disclosed by a writer of a well-known periodical called the "Presbyterian," which reveals facts that are alarming: Out of 49,-000,000 young people in the United States 36,000,000 of them have never set foot inside any church, of any creed. This same writer in another survey, learned from questionnaires sent to 55,000 children of school age, 16,000 of them had never heard of the Ten Commandments, let alone quote the Lord's prayer.

FASTING FOR CHILDREN

Fasting is beneficial to children. When a child becomes ill, very often several meals or several days fasting will fix up everything. Many children as they grow and eat rich foods, develop a pimply complexion. The source of the condition comes from the stomach to the blood and it trys to unloosen its poisonous material to some extent in the skin. Only a few days of fasting will eradicate all traces of the symptom. If proper eating is undertaken, it should not return. Scores of minor and major ailments of young people could be whipped by a short fast. Girls would not find it necessary to wear "make-up" if they would fast and pray more. A natural, healthy complexion would be the result.

Babies quite frequently suffer from over-feeding rather than under-feeding. If one considers how small a baby is and analyzes the great quantity food that is given to him in proportion to the adult, one would find it very enormous. Adults would have to drink twenty one quarts of milk daily in equivalent to a baby's feeding. The "colic," "gases in the stomach," "belching," "vomiting, "diarrhea," and many other baby disturbances can quickly be eliminated by a fast of one or more meals.

FASTED 40-DAYS—SEES MIGHTY DETROIT REVIVAL

At nineteen years of age I was dying with the flu. My temperature was 106 degrees. It was on this death bed that I surrendered completely to God. I promised the Lord I would preach the Gospel if He would heal me. Then I was caught up into heaven for twelve hours. When I came back I was perfectly healed, ready to work for Him who raised me up so miraculously. Praise His name!

Even at that young age, God said, "If I would be faithful in fasting and praying, He would raise up workers all over the world in their own tongues." He also gave me Mark 10:29-30 as a call to travel and do exploits in His name. I was shown many other things as I started my life with fastings and praying like Paul. Many times my fastings were from three days to a week and longer. In some of my fasts the Lord gave me much revelation concerning the time we live. While on a two weeks fast I cried and prayed until Jesus became so real that He appeared in my room one night. This was in the beginning of my Christian experience. The room was all lighted up, brighter than the sun. Jesus stood at the foot of my bed and a light much brighter than the sun was around Him. This great experience was very impressive and for a long time it seemed I was walking on air. Shortly after that, while fasting five days, the Lord filled me with a peculiar experience. A Roman missionary told me I was speaking a message, glorifying and praising the Lord in his language and I never did speak Italian before. It must have been the Holy Spirit talking. The missionary interpreted what I was saying.

After giving up my job, I went on a partial fast for three months, eating only once a day. The Lord gave me intercession for souls.

After praying and fasting seven days to see sinners converted and to ask the wonderful Lord to give me more of Him, the Lord sent a revival meeting to Dayton, Ohio where the Lord healed a multitude of sick folk and converted many souls. My prayer was also answered in another way when a lady gave me Dr. Franklin Hall's book on fasting and prayer. This deeper fasting experience was what I wanted. I was now able to fast longer than a week or two. I was so burdened for sinners and their bodies to be healed that I could hardly sleep at nights. With my longer fasting I could get greater victories for my intercession. I could see what God would do when multitudes would begin to fast. Jesus showed me that before long there would be workers all over the world who would fast and travail for souls. This would bring great revivals, yes greater than the world has ever seen, even greater than when Jesus was here. If it were not for this Word, it would seem unbelievable in the natural, "The works that I do shall ye do also; and greater works than these shall ye do; because I go unto my Father." John 14:12.

After fasting forty days without food and with Jesus to strengthen me, I saw many more miracles and demonstrations of the Holy Spirit. I saw the "dry bones" of Ezekiel take life. As I continued to agonize and weep for lost souls, the spirit of heaviness was upon me to such an extent, it seemed my spirit would leave the body. I saw thirty thousand souls appear before me finding Christ as their Saviour in a coliseum in Detroit, Michigan. (SINCE THIS REVELATION TO BROTHER BARTH WE UNDERSTAND THERE HAS COME TO DETROIT SOME MIGHTY HEALING-SALVATION-OUTPOURINGS, through Sister Beal, Brother Wm. Branham, Brother T. Osborn, Brother G. Lindsay, Brother F. Bosworth and Dr. Chas. Benham.) I saw another 10,000 find Jesus in an open field. Many churches, auditoriums and big tents were packed. A mighty revival is coming through fasting and prayer, but I was shown how the wealthy Laodicean churches were dealt out judgment. Their false leaders were given the judgment of Ananias and Sapphira, when they lied to the Holy Spirit.

When I was reading Brother Hall's books on fasting, the sweetest incense came down from heaven setting a seal of approval upon them. They present a teaching of Jesus Christ that if followed will truly bring a world revival among dying and lost humanity. I believe this is Jesus Christ's truth and it is the message of the hour for cold, sleepy and backslidden Christians.

Your Brother in Christ,
Leonard Barth 1776 Cherry St. Youngstown 8, Ohio

METHODIST MINISTER GETS CHURCHES REVIVED

Dear Brother Hall:

I am a Methodist minister who received your book two years ago.

After fasting and praying ten days for a revival in three Methodists churches that I am in charge of, God stirred and sent revivals in our midst. The Lord richly blessed us in many ways. A Roman Catholic and his protestant wife were among those gloriously saved.

In one of my churches a lady, (who was Italian) and to whom I gave one of your books, went on a fast of twenty-three days for her old Catholic mother who came from the old country, was blind, about to die. She was praying to beads and images. She became interested in Jesus and learned how to pray to the Lord. Finally she became gloriously saved.

The lady who fasted twenty-three days was hopelessly afflicted with kidney stones. The Doctor could do nothing for her, and said an operation would be necessary. Well praise the Lord she has not had an attack since her fast two years ago.

Before I became acquainted with fasting, my people said, "we have never heard of fasting." I said, "bless your heart, have you never read your Bible?"

Pray for as I work in these Methodist churches and kindly send a good supply of pamphlets on fasting.

Yours in Him,
R. B. Krape Woodbine R F D No. 1, Eldora, N. J.

Dear Brother Hall:

This is my first major fast, although I have eaten lightly and missed meals many times in my life for the glory of God

As I was pressing on into this fast and planning on breaking it four weeks had expired when the Lord took me into such a wonderful dream. This gave me a new grip, brought more fervor and zeal into my life and made me have a new vision of spiritual things. So impressive was this dream that I was enabled to press on and fast forty days without any food.

I do thank God for these experiences which have drawn me closer to God and given me a burden for the lost.

May God bless you,
(Mrs.) R. Clarke 3343 Patterson Ave. New Westminster B. C., Canada

Chapter IV

JESUS' FAST

The three men most highly developed spiritually are those who fasted forty days. One was the Son of God, the other two are Moses and Elijah. Other folk of great importance and high spirituality that fasted during long periods when they were under great mental strain and tribulation, are Anna the prophetess, David, Daniel, John the Baptist, and Paul. A close study of their lives shows they gained great spiritual strength, by fasting and prayer, that otherwise they would not have received.

Fasting was a part and parcel of the very life of Christ, and a very essential part that has been ignored as if it were an unsolved mystery. This was never meant to be hidden, and never should have been so overlooked. This may explain why we have not had a more complete outpouring of the latter rain. Surely such a stupendous truth cannot continue to be a secret hidden in plain sight for over nineteen hundred years. The strides and progress of man in other channels have been so enlightening and progressive. Surely we feel that it is time, and time past due for all to "Labour for Christ", in whom are all the treasures of wisdom and knowledge. Try this truth that gives such a treasure house of riches and strength.

How much did Jesus realize that He was the Son of God? He knew that He was the Son of God, but that fullest realization and illumination may not have obtained to its highest degree until after His fast, then there could not be the least shadow or faintest particle of doubt but what He became the Incarnate Son of God, the "Logos." His faith then, overcame all obstacles and doubts and was as perfect as God, Himself.

We are not told in Matthew, chapter four, the reason of His fast. It was not time for anyone to know the reason then, but in Matthew, chapter seventeen, Jesus explained it. Before this time His disciples were not able to bear this teaching. The great revelation of why He fasted was shown when He healed this lunatic boy, and answered the question that the disciples had asked him. "Why could not we cast him out!" Matt. 17:19.

It seemed that the disciples had become a reproach or disgrace to Christ because they could not heal this individual. They apparently were ashamed of themselves so they came to Jesus secretly, to ask of Him the reason why they were not able to cast out the demons. Then the secret of Jesus' fast was revealed and showed them and us what *"Super-Atomic Power"* one can have. Anyone can have that power, Thank the Lord. All can who will follow through the instructions given by Him.

"Have Faith as a grain of mustard seed . . . . and nothing shall be impossible unto you . . . . by prayer and fasting." Matt. 17:20, 21.

When Jesus declared that His faith was the product of prayer and fasting we may feel sure that He understood it to be necessary in order to express faith, as He did, in attitude, words and works. His entire life was a definition of faith in every circumstance of life. If therefore, other benefits are obtained by fasting and prayer, we may feel assured that He obtained them.

No one could give help to this major prayer problem except One. That Person had fasted forty days and forty nights, and the only one in the midst that had this great experience was none other than Jesus. (Praise His Name.)

However, Jesus clearly shows us that anyone who had had a prayer and fasting experience, could do it. There is a big difference between prayer alone, and *Prayer,* combined with fasting.

The possibility of the fast being a hindrance to JESUS can not be entertained for a moment, because in all available data on fasting, there is no evidence to warrant such an assumption. On the contrary, all evidence points to the conclusion that the fast of Jesus was an aid to HIM. The benefits derived therefrom were not accidental but earnestly sought by Him and the Spirit. In that momentous struggle there was no room for chance. JESUS AVAILED HIMSELF OF THE MOST POWERFUL AID AT HIS DISPOSAL. JESUS fasted in order to obtain certain benefits, which we have seen.

Jesus fasted in order to secure His perfect faith, He urged fasting upon His disciples to remedy their weak faith, He declared that *they would fast,* and gave directions which are intended to insure to all of His followers the same benefits of fasting which He obtained. The disuse of fasting is in direct opposition to the practice, example, and the teaching of Christ. However, we can amplify our answer from the results that were obtained from many experiences.

There is no record of Christ healing the sick, or performing any miracles until after he had fasted forty days and forty nights. Then He was more fully equipped, capable, and prepared for any and all emergencies. *At this moment how much Faith have you at your disposal, to meet any obstacle?*

When Jesus was twenty-one years old the record shows He had not yet performed a miracle. At twenty-five, he still had no healings, miracles, and no manifestation of His Divine Sonship to his credit. He became twenty-six, twenty-seven, twenty-eight and twenty-nine year of age, and yet, no miracles or manifestations. Why? He had not received the fullness of the Holy Spirit, and had not spent forty days fasting. It was necessary for Jesus to be prepared and have all the spiritual equipment before He went out for His great undertakings, etc.

Satan's rage knew no bounds at the conclusion of Christ's fast and he sought ways and means to subdue Him. Christ could not have been tempted by something He did not need. Before the fast perhaps He needed more Faith to be ready to turn stones into bread. Now, Jesus could turn these stones into bread and yield to an appetite similar to the one Eve yielded to in the Garden of Eden. The answer that Jesus gave was not only an answer to Satan, but throws a challenge to all humanity. "Man shall not live by bread alone, but by every word that proceedeth out of the mouth of God." Matt. 4:4.

Jesus, at thirty years of age, only after praying and fasting forty days and forty nights, began to manifest Himself as the Son of God with all power, signs, and wonders. There was such an awakening! Fasting is the most powerful means at the disposal of every child of God. Fasting literally becomes prayer to the praying Christian, Prayer that is as different as an Atomic Bomb compared to an ordinary bomb. Prayer alone is like the ordinary bomb, and the Fast with prayer is comparable to the Super-Atomic Bomb.

Jesus knew the positive value of prayer and fasting, and was confident that they were the only means to the end that He sought. Jesus fasted in order that prayer might become prayer in the highest sense—might reach its highest intensity. He blazed the way that we are to follow. Although Jesus knew He was the Son of God, this assurance was stamped more indelibly upon Him by the prayer and fasting of forty days.

Satan was not too much interested in Christ until He was ready to MANIFEST HIS SONSHIP. Then and only then, after His forty day fast, was Satan right on the job, ready to assail Him in every way that he could. If Christ was immune and could not have sinned or yielded to Satan at this time, then this would have been the greatest farce that the world has ever seen. Surely, Christ could have yielded to this temptation, Satan knew that He could and set about to try Him. Jesus Christ, with fasting back of Him, was well prepared for the attack. We are so thankful that although Jesus was tempted and tried in every manner, as we are, yet He did not yield to temptation, He victoriously overcame Satan.

Fasting and praying, then, aids us in overcoming temptations and trials.

When we fast and pray, we should never lose sight of the fact that our FAST must be for THE GLORY OF GOD, that Jesus shall continually have ALL PRAISE, HONOR, AND GLORY. A continual PRAISE, along with our PRAYERS, SHOULD ALWAYS BE IN OUR HEARTS TO OBTAIN THE FULLEST SPIRITUAL RESULTS. In other words, make it a time of FASTING AND PRAISE FOR THE GLORY OF GOD. Jesus, our MEDIATOR, is the ONE WHO WILL SEE THAT WE ARE RICHLY REWARDED. THE ONE WHO "BOUGHT US WITH HIS OWN BLOOD" IS CERTAINLY WORTHY OF MUCH PRAISE AND HONOR. A PRAISE THAT CONTINUALLY FLOWS FROM THE HEART IS NOT MONOTONOUS. The four beautiful LIVING CREATURES of Rev. 4:8, "REST NOT DAY AND NIGHT, SAYING, HOLY, HOLY, HOLY, LORD GOD ALMIGHTY, WHICH WAS, AND IS, AND IS TO COME." This would of course sound very foolish to the sinner, but to the Child of God it sounds like, "HALLELUJAH!" AMEN.

THREE REASONS WHY PRAYERS ARE NOT ANSWERED

1. "Ye have not, because ye ask not." Jas. 4:2.

Some folks pray, and think that they are praying, but their prayer is so weak that it doesn't even reach the ceiling of the room they are in. This limits God and makes it impossible for Him to grant us His highest blessings. We have to mean business with Christ and pray the prayer of intensity. Fasting intensifies the power of prayer.

2. "Ye ask, and receive not, because ye ask amiss, that ye may consume it upon your lusts." Jas. 4:3.

After praying earnestly and sincerely about an object, the Lord certainly will reveal to you whether or not it is His will. Form a definite decision about it once you know that it is "His Will," and go after it with your whole body, soul, and spirit and seek Him with your whole heart and "HE will be found." We must always establish ourself on the definite will of God as pertaining to our requirements. Then we go after it with all our heart without doubting.

Divine HEALING is DEFINITELY the Lord's will for us. Why try to get well in the natural if it is not HIS will? Start praising Jesus for healing.

The second reason leads us into the next.

> 3. *"This kind can come forth by nothing, but by prayer and FASTING."* Mark 9:29.

If your prayer is not answered, then go into prayer and fasting. Remember, you have not sought the Lord with your "WHOLE HEART," until you go on a protracted FAST AND PRAY. Your prayer will then be intensified so greatly that YOU WILL REALLY BE "ASKING" and you will KNOW DEFINITELY HOW MUCH IT IS THE WILL OF GOD FOR THAT OBJECT TO BE GIVEN YOU. Sickness and suffering are the works of the Devil and Jesus came to undo them, He wants to HEAL YOU NOW. If these three methods are used results cannot fail to materialize. The greatest key to this success is reason No. 3, but a like promise is given in Matt. 17. "NOTHING SHALL BE IMPOSSIBLE UNTO YOU . . . BY PRAYER AND FASTING." Do not dilly-dally around and procrastinate about it, TRY IT OUT AND SEE. THIS IS IMPORTANT. (For more details here see Joel 2:12-15).

REVIVAL IN SOUTH AFRICA AFTER FASTING 40 DAYS

1150 Pretorius St.
Pretoria, South Africa

Dear Brother Hall:

Mrs, R. Retief gave me your books on fasting to read. After I had read them I was convinced that your teaching was right. I started to fast on the 27th of May and started to break the fast on the 6th of July—thus having fasted forty days.

I had fasted before for a day or two and I thoroughly believe in it. I have been practicing the healing message too. The 40-day fast did not unduly inconvenience me. I became weak at the end after losing 38 pounds. I sought glory for my Lord through consecration. The fullness of the Holy Spirit, the conversion of the people who come to the place where I have oversight was desired and received. Several families were converted and I received money to pay my debts. My eyes that were bothering me were improved . . .

Just after the fast I spoke to a Women's Association upon "REVIVAL" through fasting and prayer. Now several of the women are fasting two days a week for a revival in this country.

The next Sacrament in our church after my fast was the largest it had been for eight years of my ministry . . . I praise the Lord that fasting will do more than prayer without fasting.

Will you and your band pray that I will always keep in His will.

Yours in Him,
J. Keith Craig

Chapter V

ONE HUNDRED REASONS WHY WE SHOULD FAST

I do not need to fast. I am too thin. You won't catch me starving myself to death. I get too weak. I am too lazy to fast. It is ridiculous to think the Lord expects me to fast. I will never fast unless the Lord puts a fast on me." These and other remarks are made by folk who have practically no understanding at all as to what fasting is all about. Only narrow minded folk and fanatics condemn something they know nothing about. If you should be one who has never fasted ten continuous days in your lifetime and never received light on the *power* and revival force of protracted fasting, why not be open minded enough to search the Bible and its facts to see for yourself, and not ignore such a major teaching as is taught in the Word of God? The practice of this message is now helping to bring a World Revival before Jesus comes.

In our evangelistic tours where we have had the privilege to contact thousands of Christians from many different denominations, we have yet to find more than several folk in a city who have ever heard or read one single complete sermon on the subject. (Two years later, we find this condition changing.)

Again, some are inclined to believe that fasting may have only one or two small virtues. Maybe it is beneficial to rid heavy folk of their fat, or the suffering one goes through its like penance and the denial of food blesses the Lord by our sacrifices.

A number of reasons are given here showing the importance of consecrated *fasting to Jesus*:

1. Fasting becomes prayer to the praying Christian. "I humbled my soul with fasting; and my prayer returned unto my bosom." Psalm 35:13.
2. Fasting takes one into humility.
3. Fasting removes pride.
4. Fasting intensifies the POWER OF PRAYER.
5. Fasting amplifies the power of prayer.
6. Fasting reaches and obtains what prayer cannot alone. Matt. 17:17-21.
7. Fasting REMOVES UNBELIEF. Matt. 17:20, 21.
8. Fasting is the greatest FAITH PRODUCER. Matt. 17:21.
9. Fasting is more closely related to FAITH THAN ANY OTHER CHRISTIAN WORK.
10. Fasting is the very threshold of FAITH, but because it is not understood it is frequently overlooked.
11. Fasting will "BLITZKRIEG" the devil.
12. Fasting is the speediest method known to spiritual success.
13. Fasting brings one face to face with reality.
14. Fasting brings one into direct contact with UNBELIEF," so that it can be removed. Unbelief can never be fully comprehended until one fasts ten to forty days.
15. Fasting masters the old man, and gives him a powerful beating.

16. Fasting pleases the spirit. "THE FLESH AND THE SPIRIT ARE AT ENMITY WITH EACH OTHER."

17. Fasting subjugates the flesh.

18. Fasting mortifies the flesh.

19. Fasting will mortify one's members. Col. 3:5.

20. Fasting is hard on the flesh, therefore it pleases Jesus. It prevents the flesh from going into a raid.

21. Fasting is the most spiritual process to bring a revival.

22. Fasting leaves the natural and takes one quickly into the spiritual realm.

23. Fasting will undo the sins of intemperance.

24. Fasting will crucify the flesh and break bad habits.

25. Fasting is self chastisement and will prevent many chastisements of the Lord from coming upon us.

26. Fasting, when properly entered into, is the surest method of consecration and sanctification.

27. Fasting is the easiest way for backsliders to come home. Study David.

28. Fasting slows down carnality and un-natural desires.

29. Fasting places our natural appetites in a dormant condition, thus physical pleasures are not enjoyed. With pleasurable appetites static, God can come near us and we near Him. He is contacted. A revival begins.

30. Fasting brings one nearer to Christ than any other known process.

31. Fasting will see our unanswered prayers answered. "Nothing shall be impossible unto him . . . by PRAYER AND FASTING." Matt. 17:21.

32. Fasting changes one's environment from the natural to the SPIRITUAL. A revival of power in the spirit is also begun.

33. Fasting sees a life of defeat transformed into a life of VICTORY; thus giving HEALING and new life to both the body and the soul.

34. Fasting develops the fruit of the Spirit and assists one in receiving spiritual gifts.

35. Fasting consumes and burns out the very roots of fleshly lusts.

36. Fasting brings one into the misery and sufferings of the fleshly nature in such a manner that one can see himself in the same light that Jesus sees him. Our unworthiness is brought into reality.

37. Fasting gives the child of God spiritual manifestations.

38. Fasting will always give one the proper anointing for work.

39. Fasting always brings revelations and better understanding of the Bible. Sometimes visions and unspeakable glory will also be manifested.

40. Fasting enlarges our capacities. Many of us have only a thimble-size capacity. We might be full at times, but how full? Shouting and spiritual emotion does not always indicate how large our capacities are. A person may be running over with only a thimble-size capacity. Fasting will give a bushel and a well-size capacity to enjoy the riches of heaven, glory and power. We then can receive rewards, depending on how long and how properly we fast and pray.

41. Fasting neutralizes the flesh so that the individual becomes a conductor of spiritual power.

42. Spiritual efficiency is highly accelerated through the fast so the in-

dividual, being a more efficient conductor to spiritual forces, likewise becomes a powerful conductor to the *healing power* of Christ; whether for his personal body or for the needs of others. Vital spiritual forces pour through individuals who have been in fastings, often.

43. Spiritual forces flowing through fasting people cause them to become more receptive to the spiritual gifts that are being poured forth today.

44. Fasting, places the candidate's sense faculties in a position so they cannot war against faith. Faith springs forth more readily and the vital contact is made in receiving divine healing or any other objective from Jesus.

45. Our strongholds of the flesh are pulled down so that faith has no real barriers. II Cor. 10:3-5. Fasting casts down reasonings so that we will not listen to the evidence that our senses may bring forth, but we let faith loose.

46. Unbelief takes its greatest holiday through fasting.

47. Fasting being a spiritual process, we learn how to believe that God will do what He tells us He will do, and we begin doubting the flesh, unbelief and the devil, rather than God's Word any longer.

48. That which could not come about, without fasting and prayer, has come about by thousands of Christians fasting longer than at any other time since the days of Christ. As the author has predicted many times, a revival was certain to come when men and women put this vital process into practice on a large scale. Today there is strong evidence to support the fact, that the mighty evangelistic healing campaigns the world over, and thousands who are receiving spiritual gifts as never before since the time of Christ, are coming about through fasting and prayer. Not necessarily a measley fast of a few meals, but major fasts are underway by many of the saints. These major fastings are from ten to forty or more days. Many who do not understand fasting or its potency may be skeptical here.

49. Fasting is a powerful process and is similar to that of faith. Very few understand or even have much faith, although most folk desire to brag that they have. The Word of God when received in true real revelation will bring faith, but often the Word cannot be received with proper revelation unless we also carry out the Word concerning fasting, then the quickening power of God's Spirit quickens things to us by powerful revelation in such a manner that FAITH shines forth in outbursts of radiant action. We can claim in all of the promises that are applicable to us that we are burdened for.

50. Fasting is a power behind DIVINE HEALING, behind the development of the fruit and the receiving of the gifts of the Spirit. No Christian can be his best without seasons of fasting and praying.

NATURAL REASONS WHY WE SHOULD FAST

There are many, many more reasons WHY ONE SHOULD FAST. We have just touched very briefly upon the most important *SPIRITUAL REASONS*. Please remember that in the above mentioned statements, we are referring only to the CONSECRATION FAST. This is the fast dedicated to Jesus by anointing ourselves with oil, or allowing the elders in the church to do so where there is a group going on a fast. Matt. 6:17. It is a fast with much prayer, consecration and yielding to the Lord. Jesus is very much pleased and honored when we come to Him, freeing ourselves from the natural. We exalt Him to the highest. Don't worry, you will be repaid a thousand times.

We are again discussing WHY I SHOULD FAST, only this time we are considering the subject from the PHYSICAL STANDPOINT INSTEAD OF THE SPIRITUAL. Please bear in mind that any person, saved or unsaved, can receive the natural, secondary physical blessings of fasting, but only the consecrated child of God can receive the great spiritual blessings. When we go into food abstention, we give the stomach a vacation and vacate into the Spirit, then the tabernacle of the Holy Spirit goes into HOUSECLEANING. Cleanliness is Godliness. Nothing can clean up the house of the Holy Spirit more effectively and quickly than by giving our stomachs a HOLIDAY. If the physical side of fasting was all that was received by abstaining from food, it certainly would be worth fasting and people would live twenty-five to thirty-five years longer (according to health authorities). Many of God's people are committing "SLOW SUICIDE" by being continually on a three meal a day stuffing habit, not satisfied with stuffing God and FAITH out of their lives, but go right on STUFFING OUT THEIR OWN LIFE YEARS AHEAD OF TIME. They stuff HEALTH OUT AND INVITE DISEASES AND DEMONS IN. AFTER WEARING OUT ONE SET OF TEETH DIGGING THEMSELVES TO THE GRAVE, MANY SECURE ANOTHER SET TO FINISH DIGGING THEMSELVES TO DEATH.

We shall consider some of the physical reasons, "WHY FAST"—BELIEVE IT OR NOT:

51. FASTING is the greatest curative agency known.

52. Fasting is the quickest curative agency known to man.

53. When you feed a diseased body you feed the disease; fasting starves the disease.

54. Fasting rids the body of all the unwanted poisonous filth of auto-intoxication and food contamination.

55. Fasting purifies the blood stream.

56. Fasting improves the circulation. It even cleanses the blood vessels so that blood circulates all through vessels that may have heretofore been closed.

57. Fasting rests the heart, improves, prevents and overcomes heart troubles.

58. FASTING CONSERVES ENERGY. Sick people cannot get well unless there is a conservation of energy. Many times food will destroy or waste what little energy a sick individual has.

59. Fasting gives the overworked stomach a vacation as well as nearly all other parts of the body.

60. Fasting rapidly removes the cause of many diseases.

61. Fasting will cure 99% of all functional ailments.

62. Fasting quickly heals simple diseases such as boils, skin blemishes, indigestion, dyspesia, auto-intoxication, constipation (although at first the fast seems to aggravate the condition), rheumatism, fever, anaemia, poor blood, asthma, change of life and irregular periodical functions in females, restoring

to normal, most various other diseases. Long fasting will also cure most other major diseases caused by impurities within the system. Barren women are often able to have children.

63. Fasting is the greatest blood purifier known.

64. Fasting eradicates mucus, stringy ropey, fecal material and floating food particals within the body.

65. Fasting usually makes an individual stronger day by day, after ten or fifteen days of fasting.

66. The headache generally felt while fasting is a sure indication that we should FAST.

67. Fasting will remove ordinary headaches and the coffee or caffeine headache as well as the over used coffee drinking HABIT, if one does not invite it back after the fast.

68. Fasting will also eradicate tobacco, drug and drinking habits in about fifteen days or less. The roots of these habits are imbedded within the stomach. Fasting consumes these very roots.

69. A person cannot starve while fasting, only the very things that are not needed within the body are used. Some of these are poisonous, contaminated, rotten food particles that have been on the walls of the stomach for months. This very condition invites disease and DEMONS, and with fasting they are starved out.

70. Fasting is the greatest youth restorer known.

71. Regular fasting prolongs life from twenty to forty years, depending on how much and how long the fasts are.

72. Fasting will remove tumors as large as watermelons, also ulcers, cancer, and goiters, arthritis, heart trouble, nervous diseases, tobacco, alcohol, drug and other habits, and will revitalize the glands.

73. Fasting causes one to become weak because the rubbish and poisons within the body are being brought to a head like a boil; it is sorest when it is brought to a head, before the core is removed. The weakness while fasting generally disappears after the worst poisons and pollutions are removed by the housecleaning process.

74. Fasting, after two weeks, more or less, causes the breath that was so foul during the first of the fast to become clean and pure like that of a child's.

75. Fasting removes the bad taste from the mouth.

76. Fasting will so purify the skin that often the complexion becomes rosy and like a child's.

77. The older a person becomes the more often he should fast. No one becomes too old to fast. History and the Bible shows us that the men and women who fasted the most, lived the longest. Study Moses and Anna.

78. Fasting overcomes many bad habits.

79. Fasting develops patience and aids temperance.

80. Fasting overcomes and aids in the *prevention of disease.*

81. Fasting draws the intestinal tract into its normal size and overcomes and prevents colitis.

82. Fasting restores a natural, normal appetite, after the fast is broken properly. The stomach being smaller requires less food.

83. Fasting is for thin, underweight people. Many times a thin person

will point to a heavy person saying they need to fast and not realize that in most cases the thin person needs the fast more than the heavy person. The reason is very simple, THE THIN INDIVIDUAL HAS MANY TIMES SO OVERWORKED THEIR ORGANS BY OVEREATING THAT THEY ARE INCAPABLE OF PUTTING ON WEIGHT. I have seen many an under-weight person fast from two to three weeks and weigh more after breaking the fast properly than they weighed before fasting. A heavy person usually is in good enough health so that his organs can help him put on weight.

84. Fasting is a normalizing agent; it will help to restore weight to under-weight folk and aid in preventing excessive weight on overweight folk.

85. Fasting will aid in cases of insomnia, although at first *an automatic blood transfusion* is set up within the body by the blood remaining in the body from the weight that is lost. This excess blood goes through the body to bathe the organs and it enters into the head causing sleeplessness for a time. Later on, and after the fast, one finds rest and sleep easier and more refreshing.

86. Excess starches and sweets cause the body to be converted into an ALCOHOLIC FACTORY. Alcohol is manufactured from them, this in turn causes HABIT HUNGER which is LUST HUNGER and it is entirely different than true hunger. There are perhaps more people bound to this habit than there are to the drinking habit. The former is about as difficult to break. Jesus classifies it just as much of a sin as the DRINK HABIT. Luke 21: FASTING WILL UNDO THE HUNGER HABIT OF LUST AND WILL PREVENT FOLK FROM BEING DRUNK ON FOOD.

87. Fasting should be frequent, to clean and keep clean the temple and home of the Holy Spirit.

88. Fasting aids and improves our sight, hearing, taste, touch and smell. All sense faculties are benefited.

89. Fasting improves the mental faculties, making it easier to think, study, remember and concentrate more efficiently. (During some parts of the fast, at first, this may not always be true.)

90. Fasting seems to take one into a different world. It is wonderful to taste and experience. It makes for better harmony for the person, his family, friends and community.

91. Fasting is a tremendous power, whether it is used for God or our-selves. Individuals, whether Christians or not, who have fasted for their career, vocation, skill or "labors," will have results. But when a fast is per-formed for this purpose, the Scripture informs us we will not have our Father's reward. We may have our own reward or the reward of man. ("In the day of your fast ye find pleasure, and EXACT YOUR LABOURS." Isaiah 58:3, 4. Also Matt. 6:16-18).

92. If heathen people in other lands fast many days and many weeks to demons and the devil, and by their fastings are able to do exploits. They attribute their power to their fasting to these spirits. And many times these exploits are miraculous and of greater power than many Christians are able to do without fasting. How much more could the Children of God accom-plish to perform the supernatural through fasting and prayer. It puts us to shame when we think of multitudes of suffering and dying humanity.

93. Fasting is a tremendous invisible force, natural as well as spiritual,

whether used for God, our self or Satan. We should recognize this value, but we should be the more willing to fast for Jesus.

94. According to some Christian Physicians, there is no habit or weakness that can survive a siege of fasting and prayer.

95. Fasting enables one to conquer self desires and habit of masturbation. Col. 3:5 and Rev. 2:7.

96. One of the worst habits, but it is not looked upon as such a bad habit, because it excuses itself under the good name of good food, is nothing more than the *stuffing habit*. A surfeiter is placed ahead of the drinker. Luke 21:34 and see Matthew 24th Chapter. Fasting breaks this habit also.

97. A good thing is disguised in order to give a front and an excuse for the indulgence in same. Satan delights in having God's people sin in a way that they think it is not sin. There is a record in God's word of more people destroyed at one time from over eating than from getting drunk with alcoholic drinks, believe it or not. (Read Psalm 78.) The biggest sin of our Lord's people is their continued stuffing His Spirit and power out from their lives so they will become self-righteous. This is one of the contributing causes of self-righteousness. This habit often leads to worse habits such as the alcoholic habit. The next thing following self-righteousness is that the individual becomes bound to some denomination or preacher. If the preacher does not follow God's pattern properly the follower also is led astray, oftentimes being led into false doctrines. Rom. 16:17-18. With the oil lost from their lamps they become the class of foolish virgins the Bible speaks about when Jesus returns. Fasting is a certain remedy for this.

98. Fasting not only keeps our natural appetites subdued, but the natural appetite of eating is mastered from habit hunger, so that we eat what we need instead of what we lust after.

99. Fasting is the ladies' best beautifier; it brings grace, charm and brings into normalcy all female functions. (While on the fast they may become abnormal).

100. Fasting is the best method for self control in all things. This applies to our mental faculties, anger, impatience, nervousness, and restlessness.

A world-wide revival will surely begin as saints of God take up the burden of the travailing prayer of fasting. Please send in names and addresses and free sermons and literature will be mailed to them.

CANADIAN FASTS FORTY DAYS IN ZERO WEATHER

Dear Brother Hall:

Greetings in Jesus name. I am just breaking my 40-day fast and realy feel fine. Praise God I was never hungry during the whole fast. I felt fine all the time and was always up and around inside and outside where the temperatures have been below zero this winter here in Saskatchewan.

I was fasting and praying for a revival among the saints of God.

I feel this has been the greatest experience of my life and many bondages has been broken in my life. I have freedom that I never have had before. Please send me the following tracts ....

Thanking you, I remain

Dave W. Siggelkow, 708 19th Street, West,, Saskatoon, Sask., Canada

DAVID'S FAST

All Christians are delighted to read the Psalms; they encourage us to press onward, and there are scores of promises and blessings for believers. The Psalms are a product of Fasting and Prayer. The sublime utterances in the Psalms are not exaggerations, as have been asserted by some, and only in the higher receptivity are made possible. Only by prayer and fasting is the soul able to receive these revelations. Read Psalms 35:13; 69:10, Psalm 78:18-32; 107:17-18 and 109:22-26, (II Sam. 12:16-23).

David sought God in long fasts; in fact he fasted so long at times that he looked like a skeleton. Psalms 109:23. "I am tossed up and down as the locust. My knees are weak through fasting; and my flesh faileth of fatness. I became a reproach unto them: when they looked upon me they shaked their heads." So much fat was lost that he actually became a reproach to look at; his friends and neighbors shook their heads. No doubt some ceased to be his friends and began criticizing; this is just what happens today when an individual seeks GOD far enough in fasting and prayer. Some people say we should always go into the desert or wilderness to fast like Moses and Christ. That is good, but here is an instance where David didn't care who saw him.

David must have fasted forty days or longer to have lost so much weight. David wasn't intersted about how he appeared, he went into it in mourning and humbleness; he was only interested in how he could please God and reach HIM. I have seen many folk who fasted longer than forty days and looked better than this description of David.

As certainly as we "labor for the meat above," we shall not stand in very high favor with the world. When we enter into the spirit of fasting and prayer, we actually are not interested in what others say about us. We are after that which is worth more than silver and gold. If you fast and pray, really get into the spirit of it, your prayers will seem more difficult at times, even than when you are praying without fasting. The main victories usually are attained after fasting.

The reason for this is that you are progressing further, reaching higher mountains to climb, darker places to penetrate, higher walls to surmount, deeper depths to plow through, etc. (See Chart No. VI, Hindrances and Obstacles). Psalm 35:13: "I humbled my soul with FASTING; and my PRAYER RETURNED INTO MY BOSOM." Fasting isn't something to glory in or to be puffed up about. Along with the fast we are to go down, into humility, disregard what people think and say. It should be a time of real weeping and mourning. Our unworthiness should be realized and the farther down we go the higher up our Christian experience will be. It will be a great spiritual fight all the way through.

I wish to state that some children of the Lord fail to press into the proper place of prayer, along with the fast, just because they find it difficult to pray; however, that is no reason for not praying. Your prayers will absolutely blast through to heaven if you settle down to doing it, and "Labor" at it as Jesus asked us to do. The Devil will be around to hinder and prevent you from accomplishing your purpose, but PRAY THROUGH, FAST THROUGH and pray until you open heaven; and continue to do this. Shorter prayers under the influence of fasting are far more effective than long prayers off the fast. We are in a channel of prayer—while fasting—that can't otherwise be possible.

Usually, the first few days of a fast are the most difficult to pray because the weakness of the body has not left, and the body has not been cleansed. Pray as much as possible, as long as possible, as fervently as possible, regardless of lack of strength and when you get over "THE HUMP" it becomes easier to fast and, generally speaking you get stronger physically. You can gradually put yourself into it, devoting more time to the prayer; then the fast itself actually becomes prayer. Please bear this in mind when fasting. A Christian then has such power that these obstacles mentioned will seem easier and easier to surmount, one presses on to more and greater obstacles all of which will be victoriously overcome, and a continually greater power than ever be left with the person as long as the individual stays in the center of God's will.

Again, I shall emphasize that prayer with the fast is very important. To those who are employed or working at various places, and it is difficult to place all your time seeking God in praying in connection with the fast, you can still secure very desirable results and the Lord will bless you much if you can keep in a spirit of prayer while you work. If one's work is extremely burdensome it will be difficult to fast and to concentrate on prayer. Sometimes a person on a job has begun a fast and time of prayer, and has gotten into the spirit of it in such a way that nothing but Jesus Christ matters, they lose interest in their work and everything else around them, to such an extent they receive a special call of God in their lives.

Some years ago, a shoe cobbler did this very thing. He was living in Denver, Colo. After fasting and praying for forty days, the power of God became so real and precious that he gave up his shoe business and went to the street corners and started blessing people through his ministry for Christ. Hundreds of sick people were prayed for daily and many were healed. Blind eyes were opened; deaf ears were unstopped; deaf and dumb spoke; ulcers, cancer, arthritis, and tuberculosis cases were healed. The lame leaped for joy. Wheel chairs, beds, crutches and braces were left behind by the ones that were healed in Jesus' name. All this in answer to the prayers of an individual who caught a revelation through prayer and fasting for forty days.

Every minister owes it to his congregation to be his best; every evangelist owes it to his revival that is being conducted; every teacher owes it to his pupils; every Christian to his brethren to be at his best spiritually; and we have seen that this is impossible without prayer and fasting. Prayer becomes illuminated and fasting makes prayer as powerful as dynamite in its results.

SHOULD I WAIT FOR GOD TO LAY A FAST BURDEN UPON ME?

No, not necessarily, for the simple reason, if we waited for God to lay a prayer burden upon us, there probably would be no praying or very little. Fasting is like praying. We fast when there is a need and because it is our Christian duty. In Mark 2:20, Jesus has already laid a fast upon us.

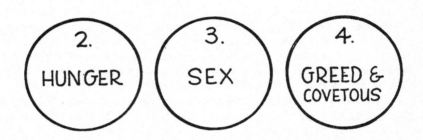

THE FOUR APPETITES BEFORE FASTING

CHART No. IV. The spiritual appetite is insignificantly developed compared with the three natural appetites. This is the way the average Christian appears to God before fasting. It explains why it is so difficult for a person to obtain the necessary SPIRITUAL PROGRESS in their life without the natural carnal appetites being subdued first. Fasting is the key and almost the only process that guarantees the complete conquering and mastering of self and the desire nature for a time so the complete manifestation of the power of God will be made available. "NOTHING SHALL BE IMPOSSIBLE BY PRAYER AND FASTING." The body is the servant of the soul. Fasting masters this body; God comes within our reach and Heaven is opened.

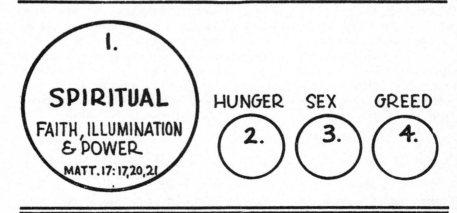

THE FOUR APPETITES DEPICTED AFTER FASTING

CHART No. V. Note that the spiritual appetite is highly active and developed at the conclusion of a protracted fast compared to the appetites of HUNGER, SEX, and GREED (covetousness). The love of food is "THE SECOND ROOT OF ALL EVIL." In a major fast HUNGER IS ABOLISHED after several days and with it every desire of Sex and later on Greed, all NATURAL DESIRES LEAVE and as far as the faster is concerned, he has none, then and only then can an individual be receptive and empty enough to receive the greater things and spiritual gifts of God which come to us by FAITH. Prayer becomes intensified, fasting becomes prayer and the individual reaches a spiritual height with God that is possible in no other way. "God is a Spirit and they that worship Him must worship Him in Spirit and Truth." Jn. 4:24. For more details here, see the author's 224 page text book on subject, "THE FASTING PRAYER." Many illustrations show how this works.

Chapter VI

THE FOUR APPETITES

Humanity is confronted with four appetites. One or more of these major appetites can get the best of us, if we allow them to do so. Intemperance and extreme indulgence can be entered into regarding them. The Bible admonishes us to be "Temperate in all things." The four appetites are:

1. THE SPIRITUAL APPETITE
2. THE HUNGER APPETITE.
3. THE APPETITE OF SEX.
4. THE APPETITE OF GREED. (Covetousness)

Please notice the charts on same.

The appetite of hunger is what will be discussed mostly under this heading. It holds the key to all the others. Food stimulates both sex and greed.

The lust of sin can be gratified in one or more of these appetites. Three of these appetites are carnal or worldly, while one is our religious or spiritual nature. Even sinners have a spiritual or religious nature, regardless of whether or not that sinner serves the true and living God.

It was through yielding to temptation that Eve gave way to satisfying her "desire" nature, gratifying these same appetites. The temptation of Jesus Christ was similar to that of Eve's temptation, and it was exactly these same four appetites that Satan chose to tempt Jesus. Namely: Hunger—"Command that these stones be made bread." Matt. 4:3-10.

The spiritual appetite intercepts all the natural appetites by the way and manner that these are gratified, whether for good or evil.

Did Jesus please Satan and yield to the appetite of hunger to use his spiritual power—spiritual appetite to perform a miracle?

Sex appetite—when a person tries to commit suicide or kill another or tempts God along the line of suicide or murder, we find that it is related to the sex nature, as sex and death, or life and death are kindred. Through our creative forces God gives us life and health, and also our offspring that we love.

The ancients, the Magi, and the wise men of the Bible so considered the creative forces of man as related to death. They, too, knew that an individual with an irrational sex nature sometimes had a suicidal mania and also that it was one of the contributing causes to lusty, bloody crimes of torture and killing. The life giving forces of nature can be used for a blessing or for destructive purposes.

In the zodiacal sign, "Scorpio," which is the eighth sign, we have a picture of a scorpion with its stinger lifted ready to strike. This is the sign of death and is supposed to govern the sex area. Just before this sign in the heavens, there is a sign of the Judge, Jesus, who is the giver of LIFE. Jesus proceeds toward death and pulls the STING OUT OF DEATH. "Oh, death, where is thy sting, oh, grave, where is thy victory."

Likewise, today among students it is generally understood that the creative forces of man are kindred to both life and death in the natural. However, it is not difficult for any of us to understand that the proper care of the creative physical forces of man leads to long life and the improper abuse of them is a speedy way to the grave.

When Satan tempted Christ, "Then the devil taketh Him up into the Holy City, and setteth Him on a pinnacle of the temple and saith unto Him, if thou be the Son of God, cast Thyself down: for it is written, He shall give His angels charge concerning Thee: and in their hands they shall bear thee up, lest at any time thou dash thy foot against a stone," Matt. 4:5, 6, Satan's rage knew no bounds. Jesus Christ was now coming into the full manifestation of His sonship. The manifestation of the Son of God. He was now prepared to begin His ministry. He had the victory that He sought. Satan had previously failed to destroy Christ when He was a baby, through King Herod; now Satan sought to get rid of Him and ruin Him by these temptations. Satan was trying to get Christ to do something foolish; this temptation could have been a way towards a suicidal destruction of Christ. No! Satan did not destroy Jesus here. Jesus did not yield to this temptation. This would have satisfied the "Desire" nature of the appetite, "Sex" (No. 3), of the appetites.

It is very important for the reader to have these four appetites fixed in his mind firmly, because all of these appetites are influenced one way or another in or out of fasting. A close understanding of them will enable one to have a richer knowledge of the Bible and of the purpose of fasting. A much more vivid understanding of the whole temptation of Christ will be seen. We are also tempted thru these same appetites.

The covetous appetite of GREED, which is No. 4, was perhaps Satan's trump card. His greatest offer to Christ was to "show Him all the Kingdoms of the world, and the glory of them; and saith unto Him, all these things will I give thee if thou wilt fall down and worship me." Matt. 4:8, 9.

The appetite of covetous greed is an appetite of abnormal desire. Desire for posessions, property, money, wealth, power, and—desire for any kind of worldly possession, even clothes. These desires, placed above our love for God, make the covetous appetite sin.

All of these appetites are normal in their proper places. Here, as in the other two major temptations, Satan was calling on Jesus to utilize His Spiritual appetite; this time to worship Satan himself, in exchange for the kingdoms and power of wealth. Many, sad to say, have sold out to worldly possessions.

The possession of these kingdoms and power would lead to the gratification of the desire—of greed. He could have had possession of these kingdoms had He yielded to the greed nature. This, thank the Lord, He did not do—Satan was badly defeated.

Satan did have it in his power, then and now, to offer Christ the kingdoms of this world, because now he is "the god of this world." Satan is a usurper. His power will not be for long. In Revelation 5:7, we see Jesus getting up from the right hand of the Father and taking the title deed of the world, the "book." Soon Satan will be evicted from the heavens and the earth, and then Jesus' throne will be set up. Blessed be the name of the Lord.

Thus the four appetites of man have been shown herewith so we can realize better what happens spiritually when we fast.

All Christians with everyday cares of business, job, and home, are usually so out of tune with the spiritual realm, that it seems practically impossible to get in communion with God. Therefore we are not in a position to contact God about our major problems.

Every person has these four appetites. Perhaps one or the other is more intensified in some respects—more intensified than they are shown in the chart "before fasting." But, nevertheless, whether or not we realize it, the spiritual appetite is insufficiently developed, compared to the carnal appetites of the flesh.

THREE APPETITES LEAVE

Now herein lies a WONDER that seems a miracle. After several days of the fast have passed, the hunger appetite actually leaves you. If the fast is prolonged, in a few days, possibly a week or ten days more, the weakness leaves and the average individual even feels stronger than he did before he began the fast. (It takes longer for the weakness to leave older people.)

The next thing that is noticed, and this is noticeable during the first of the fast, appetite (No. 3), sex desire leaves.

Then, finally, as the one who is fasting proceeds to pray and commune with God, and earnestly seeks the God of Heavens, the greed appetite No. 4, or the appetite that is the over anxious driving force which causes man to work at his job, home affairs, his business, becomes so diminished that it seems insignificant. GREED usually requires many days of fasting before diminishing. This explains why a long fast is sometimes necessary. The chief interest now is seeking God in prayer and fasting. One becomes indifferent about natural things. It seems wonderful that one is glorifying God in his whole body, soul, and spirit, with all of his members focused toward heaven.

So glorious an ecstasy is this marvelous experience that our every faculty can at last be extended toward heaven for the Glory of Jesus Christ. The precious Holy Spirit may at last have His way with our lives in every way and detail. We hear His voice more effectively.

If God's people could for one moment realize how tremendous a thing this fasting truth is, there would be thousands more who would fast. As a result, we would see the major miracles performed and a NATIONAL REVIVAL would occur. The dead would arise, demons would be cast out, thousands of incurable diseases healed, all in the name of Jesus. Will you do your part?

Now your attention is called to the chart—after a fast (Chart V, four appetites after fasting). See appetite No. 1 take predominance over the other appetites. Our entire nature seems to be unloosed from the clutches of the natural, and we take on a new environment. We see the Body of Christ as one. We are no longer bound.

Heavy trials and tribulations will be present, and many burdens and obstacles seem to come across our pathway. At times it seems that there is a wall against us which our prayers cannot penetrate. Do not be discouraged. If you do not give up, certain victory lies ahead. You are in a great spiritual battle.

There will be other times while praying, that it will seem as though you are in heaven, even visions and revelations from God may be yours.

Generally speaking, fasting will be a heavy, burdensome experience, because Satan does not want you to obtain the "FAITH" that is promised to one who fasts. You will be fighting against spiritual forces of darkness. Please bear in mind that to obtain the spiritual results, prayer, much prayer must continually be brought forth with the fast. "As soon as Zion travailed she brought forth children." Isa. 66:8.

Here is an interesting letter from a sister who fasted 24 days.

I wish to say that fasting is wonderful. I fasted for twenty-four days without food, drinking only water. When I was two weeks in my fast an epileptic boy that I was burdened for, the son of a friend of mine, was anointed and prayed for. Immediately we felt something leave him; they were demons; the son got up smiling and rejoicing and in a day or two he secured employment for the first time in his life and is still working today, several months later. This boy was taken to many places to be prayed for many times, including Angelus Temple. His condition was very bad before he was healed.

I continued the fast under Rev. Hall's instructions for three weeks and three days. I worked in the home, cooking three meals a day for my family and never got hungry. I felt stronger than I ever felt in many years. I walked several blocks to catch the bus to go to the Auditorium, sometimes twice daily. I am so thankful to know about fasting and prayer and can say that it helped me much both spiritually and physically. I was forced to break the fast before I intended to, due to criticism, but I thank God for answering many of my prayers.

Mrs. Mary Williams,
National City, Calif.

Another person who had been fasting claimed to have seen a vision of Christ around the boy mentioned in the above testimony.

A sister who had been fasting also reported seeing the demons leave the boy and go into the rear of the auditorium. She said they were hideous looking things.

Again we refer you to Mark 9:29 "And He said unto them, 'THIS KIND CAN COME FORTH BY NOTHING BUT BY PRAYER AND FASTING'."

Chapter VII

THE FOUR GREAT ESSENTIALS

There are four things which are necessary in order to exist in life. They are herewith placed in the order of their importance:

1. THE FIRST GREAT ESSENTIAL TO LIFE IS AIR, NOT FOOD.
2. THE SECOND IS NOT FOOD, AS SOME WOULD SUPPOSE, BUT WATER.
3. THE THIRD, IS STILL NOT FOOD, BUT SLEEP.
4. FOOD IS THE FOURTH GREAT ESSENTIAL.

Of the four great essentials food is generally put first, because we have to pay for it; while air, water and sleep are available on "when needed" basis, without cost.

For illustration, little animals, tested in the laboratories, have taught us some interesting things. These animals, deprived of food, but not water, for twenty days, lost more than half their weight, yet were saved by judicious feeding. However, when they were completely deprived of sleep, even while getting more careful feeding and other attention, they died within five days.

The human being reacts somewhat similarly. In a protracted fast, extending into weeks of time, a person can rest and sleep properly, and come out feeling fine. The longest period of authentic wakefulness on record is not quite ten days. Legends of prolonged insomnia are heard from time to time, but they have never been verified, thus they continue as mere legends; consequently, food is proven to be less important than sleep.

Food is less important than water because a man in a hot desert sun will die in a few hours, or several days at the most, if he hasn't water to drink; this is more fully explained elsewhere. Food is less important than the air we breathe, because, if we could not breathe, thereby getting fresh air into our lungs, we would die in a few moments. So food does not have as important a place in life, as most of us are inclined to believe. Although a person can continue weeks and sometimes even months without anything to eat, which is much longer than he could get along without any of the other essentials, food has a very important place in the physical welfare. Please see the chapter following this one on how long a person can fast. We have just shown how important, in their respective order, the FOUR GREAT ESSENTIALS are to the physical man. There are other essentials that far outshadow the above mentioned essentials for the SPIRITUAL SIDE OF MAN.

THE FOUR SPIRITUAL ESSENTIALS

The greatest of all ESSENTIALS for man is THE LORD JESUS CHRIST. This is ETERNAL LIFE. If we have HIM we have "THAT BREAD OF LIFE," and we have the source of all other essentials. This is the FIRST ESSENTIAL.

(2) The second great spiritual essential is the Baptism of the Holy Spirit, He is for all believers. "Have you received THE HOLY GHOST SINCE YE

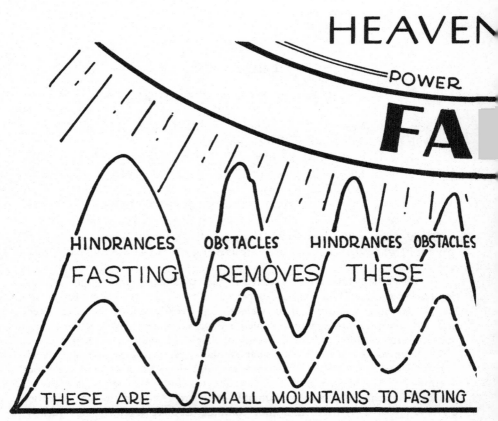

HINDRANCES OBSTACLES HINDRANCES OBSTACLES

FASTING REMOVES THESE

THESE ARE SMALL MOUNTAINS TO FASTING

CHART NO. VI. This illustrates THE BIG MOUNTAINS THAT ARE REMOVED BY "FAITH" AS REQUIRED BY FASTING AND PRAYER. They may seem very difficult by prayer alone. "HAVE FAITH AS A GRAIN OF MUSTARD SEED, YE SHALL SAY UNTO THIS MOUNTAIN, *RE-MOVE,* and IT SHALL REMOVE TO YONDER PLACE." Matt. 17:21, 22. THE RECIPE FOR THIS FAITH IS, PRAYER, FASTING and PRAISE.

BELIEVED?" (Acts 19:2.) CHRISTIANS WERE ASKED THIS QUESTION. See also Acts 11:15; 15:8, etc. This is a very important essential for the believer so that he may have the *power* that all believers need and be able to better serve the Lord. So IMPORTANT AN ESSENTIAL IS THIS TO THE CHRISTIAN THAT IT *IS* A COMMANDMENT. Acts 1:4-8.

(3) The third great essential is also from our Lord. This is Spiritual DIVINE HEALING, in answer to the prayer of FAITH. See James, chapter five. If we do not have enough FAITH to obtain our healing, it is definitely pointed out in Mark 9:29 that the reason why we do not have FAITH is because we do not FAST with our prayers. One reason FASTING is not understood is because it is very near like FAITH. It is the threshold of faith itself.

(4) The last GREAT ESSENTIAL for the believer is: JESUS MUST RETURN "SO THAT THE DEAD IN CHRIST SHALL RISE AND WE

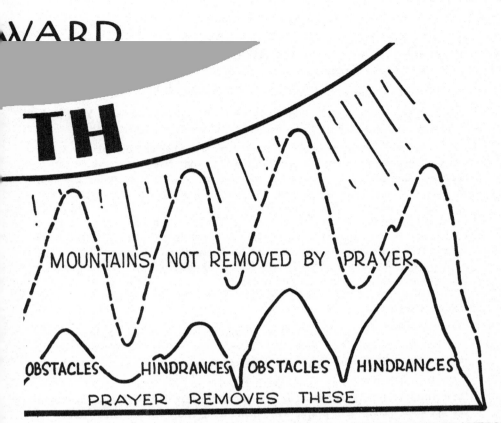

MOUNTAINS NOT REMOVED BY PRAYER

OBSTACLES   HINDRANCES   OBSTACLES   HINDRANCES

PRAYER   REMOVES   THESE

The lower mountains represent ANSWERS TO MANY OF OUR PRAYERS. THE DOTTED LINES IN BACKGROUND represent our UNANSWERED PRAYERS THAT COMETH ABOUT "BY NOTHING EXCEPT PRAYER AND FASTING." "Whosoever shall say unto this mountain, be thou removed and cast into the sea; and shall NOT DOUBT . . . He shall have whatsoever he sayeth." Mark 11:23; also Mark 9:29. Fast! Praise! Believe!

WHICH ARE ALIVE AND REMAIN SHALL BE CAUGHT UP TO-GETHER WITH THEM IN THE CLOUDS, TO MEET THE LORD IN THE AIR: AND SO SHALL WE EVER BE WITH THE LORD." I THESS. 4:17.

Before MAN can be adapted to the SPIRITUAL REALM and see Heaven, he has to BE BORN AGAIN and be like JESUS CHRIST. In the first place, you can't get to HEAVEN the way you are, because YOUR BODY IS WRONG! Supreme Intelligence designed the human body for the physical con-ditions of the planet EARTH, and it is perfect for that environment. It would be just as much out of order for worms to live in the air and birds to live in the earth as man to live in heaven without this new birth. Our bodies would be utterly useless on any other planet.

Suppose you should desire to go to the neighboring planet, MERCURY. You could not take your body there, as it is seven-tenths fluids, and water boils at 212 degrees Fahrenheit. Mercury, being so near to the sun has a temperature of 750 degrees Fahrenheit. In a couple of hours you would be buried under a stone with this inscription:

"WELL DONE! THOU GOOD AND FAITHFUL SERVANT"

Indeed you would be well done. You would be burned to a crisp. Your body would be no good on that heavenly body, because Mercury is too hot.

To illustrate further what we mean, let us see what another planet is like much farther away. It requires one hundred and sixty-five years, approximately, for the planet Neptune to make the complete zodiacal circuit around the sun; that is, one year on Neptune is one hundred sixty-five earth years. The temperature is around 400 degrees below zero, Fahrenheit! In less than thirty minutes you would be a solid block of ice, and not even the heat of Mercury could thaw you back to life again. In fact there is no other heavenly body in our solar system where your present body could remain alive. The lack of atmosphere, the absence of water and food, and the difference in temperature and gravity makes it absolutely impossible for a human body to survive off the planet Earth. How could your body occupy Heaven? Heaven lies farther beyond our solar system.

The NEW BIRTH IS THE ANSWER and some day we shall possess a body that is HEAVENLY. Our body must have a seed planted in it which is our new nature, and the new birth gives this to us.

THE FOUR GOSPELS, along with the rest of the New Testament, teach these fundamental essentials. It is also the main teaching of Jesus Christ and the apostles. Fasting and prayer will enable us to more fully realize them.

The first four essentials come to us through the FOUR ELEMENTS:

1. EARTH	3. FIRE
2. AIR	4. WATER

The second group of Spiritual essentials come to us through GOD in HIS THREEFOLD PERSONALITY PLUS THE *MAN* NATURE THAT JESUS CHRIST TOOK UPON HIMSELF SO THAT MAN COULD BE RE- DEEMED; they are.

1. GOD THE FATHER	4. GOD THE MAN
2. GOD THE SON	(THE SON OF MAN)
3. GOD THE SPIRIT	Jesus became man as well as God.

FOR A CLEARER PICTURE, please see CHARTS IX and XII, THE BODY RENOVATED (MAN DIAGRAMMED) and THE WELLS OF LIVING WATER, last chapter.

We urge you to obtain the author's book, *"Glorified Fasting"*. This is volume two of the set of four different books on subject. "Glorified Fasting" gives the "whys", "whats", "whens", and "wherefores" of Fasting. It goes completely into this subject in a different manner.

This leads us to the FOUR ESSENTIALS OF MAN (AS A CHRISTIAN):

1. BODY
2. SOUL

3. SPIRIT
4. NEW BIRTH or
   LIFE ETERNAL

THE FOUR ESSENTIALS (AS SINNERS):

1. BODY
2. SOUL

3. SPIRIT
4. D E A T H

The "Four Living Creatures" about the throne of God, a closer study of what we have just mentioned and many other fours in the Bible make a most unusual study. However this could be a volume in itself.

Chart No. VII.

TIME REQUIRED FOR HUNGER AND WEAKNESS TO LEAVE

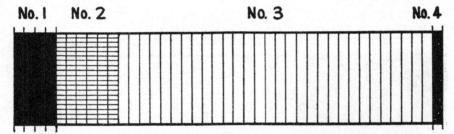

No. 1   No. 2   No. 3   No. 4

Each section represents one day

CHART SHOWING THE FOUR PHASES OF FASTING ON A 40-DAY SCALE:

1. DARK AREA: APPROXIMATE TIME REQUIRED FOR HUNGER TO LEAVE.
2. SHADED AREA: APPROXIMATE TIME REQUIRED FOR WEAKNESS TO LEAVE. (IT MAY TAPER OFF.)
3. LIGHT AREA: THE FAST PROPER; FASTING IS ROUTINE HERE, AFTER THE BODY IS CLEANSED.
4. HUNGER RETURNS AFTER A COMPLETE FAST.

Note: With different individuals the time may vary greatly in respect to the length of each phase. It may be shorter or longer. The contrast may be greater between young people and older persons. Only the approximate average is shown above.

It is more difficult for an older person to fast although they may need it more from the physical standpoint. It takes a lot longer time for the weakness to leave; sometimes fainting tendencies may be felt and due to this condition it is wise that an older person be with another individual to help him around until weakness leaves. Sometimes several fasts of a week or ten days may be better first, before a long one is undertaken.

Second: After another few days, or within a week or two, depending on the age, the weakness that you have encountered generally leaves and fasting becomes much easier. (In some instances it may be much longer).

Third: Now the fast after eight, ten or fifteen days, more or less, becomes a matter of routine and actually becomes easier. You should concentrate on efforts in prayer, an answer from heaven, a revelation, healing, or spiritual operations in your life.

CHART No. VIII.

AVERAGE AMOUNT OF EFFORT REQUIRED IN FASTING

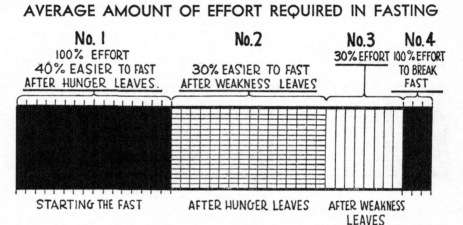

No. 1	No. 2	No. 3	No. 4
100% EFFORT		30% EFFORT	100% EFFORT
40% EASIER TO FAST	30% EASIER TO FAST		TO BREAK
AFTER HUNGER LEAVES.	AFTER WEAKNESS LEAVES		FAST

STARTING THE FAST   AFTER HUNGER LEAVES   AFTER WEAKNESS LEAVES

CHART SHOWING THE PERCENTAGE OF EFFORT REQUIRED IN TAKING A PROTRACTED FAST. (FIGURES ESTIMATED ONLY)

1. IT REQUIRES 100% EFFORT AND WILL POWER TO GET STARTED. SOMETIMES SEVERAL ATTEMPTS WILL HAVE TO BE MADE. THE FIRST DAYS ARE THE MOST DIFFICULT. Do not be discouraged if you have to make many attempts.

2. IT BECOMES EASIER TO FAST AFTER HUNGER LEAVES.

3. AFTER WEAKNESS LEAVES, FASTING BECOMES ROUTINE AND IS NOT NEARLY SO DIFFICULT.

4. IT REQUIRES AS MUCH EFFORT TO BREAK THE FAST PROPERLY AS IT DID TO BEGIN THE FAST.

For more details, please consult Author's other three books. (All books different). *"THE FASTING PRAYER," "GLORIFIED FASTING"* and *"BECAUSE OF UNBELIEF," "OUR DIVINE HEALING OBLIGATION."*

Chapter VIII

HOW TO FAST

Speaking of food, perhaps one never realizes the great quantity of food which is consumed in the course of a month by an ordinary individual, until one fasts. Most of the American people consume too much food and according to health experts, the American people as a whole suffer more or less with auto-intoxication. The scriptures show us plainly that we should be temperate in all things. A study of Psalm 78, along with other scriptures, shows us vividly how God dislikes the glutton. Here they lusted for more food while food was still in their mouths and God utterly destroyed the fattest ones.

Some people wear out one set of teeth digging their way to the grave. Then they buy a second set to finish eating themselves to death.

William Penn, the founder of Pennsylvania, has said concerning temperance: "To this a spare diet contributes much. Eat therefore to live and do not live to eat. That's like a man, but this below a beast."

It is very important to point out here for emphasis that fasting and star-vation are two entirely different things. Fasting is a phisiological process. Whereas fasting is beneficial and will rid the body of most diseases when present, starvation is detrimental, and if continued long enough, ends in death. (This seldom could ever happen before approximately a hundred days.) The difference between these two processes is fundamental.

The appetite of hunger will have to be abolished for the time being with ex-treme will power and assistance from the Lord. The first days of the fast are very, very difficult. Sometimes several attempts will be necessary before the candidate will have fasted long enough for hunger to leave. Not only does the body crave food at stated and regular times, by reason of long-continued habit, but the mind likewise becomes restless and continues to remind one that food would be relished.

One never realizes until he begins a fast how important a factor food really is—to his mental frame of mind, as well as physical and spiritual being. As long as the body is continually nourished, one does not think of food to any great extent, but as soon as it is withheld, it begins to occupy an important part in the mental life; one has a constant tendency to think of food. He antici-pates even at the very beginning of the fast, the day when abstinence will termi-nate, and when eating will again become possible. This craving of the body can be overcome only by immediate distraction and keeping in the spirit of prayer. A glass or two of water will alleviate the immediate gnawing symptoms which usually develop in the region of the stomach. These sensations are pro-duced by the rhythmic activity of the muscles in and about the stomach, and are present when food is first withheld, and when the thought of food enters the mind. As soon as this thought is banished by concentration upon Christ. these rhythmical muscular contractions (known as the *peristaltic action*) soon subside. After a little time, these acute sensations of hunger will pass away, possibly to occur again later, perhaps at the next regular meal time. A repetition of the water drinking and prompt distraction of attention will again dispose of these symptoms. After three or four days, it will be found that real hunger will not return again until the return of natural hunger at the conclusion of the fast. Habit hunger, which is different, will often come about, and leave just as unexpectedly as it came.

SALT WATER FLUSH

If one wishes to hasten the effects of fasting at the beginning, a salt water flush can be used to flush out the colon (This should NOT be done after the first several days IN THE FAST). To one quart of hot water, add two level teaspoons of salt and drink. This may be done at any other time on an empty stomach, when not fasting, for cleansing purposes.

Fasting is much easier when we see it in three dimensions. First: After several days, hunger leaves. It is then a step easier to fast. See Chart VII.

Prayer in the consecration fast cannot be over-emphasized. Intense prayer positively must accompany the fast if the spiritual results as stated are to be obtained in the fullest measure as desired.

Very often during a fast one will become highly sensitive to the taste of water. The taste sense becomes very acute, as well as all of the senses, and one will detect flavors and metallic tastes never tasted before. Bottled or other pure water is preferable to ordinary hydrant water.

To avoid cramps in the stomach and some other unpleasantness, hot or warm water should be drunk instead of cold water, unless the cold water is taken very, very slowly. This is more important if a person is thin or a fast taken in cold weather.

One of the greatest obstacles which must be overcome by practically all those who undertake this unusual beneficial experience will be the persuasion of over-solicitous relatives and friends who invariably endeavor to tempt the patient to break his fast prematurely, under the impression that he is injuring his body, or he is starving to death. These persuasions of over-solicitous relatives become very strong and insidious and he may fall by the wayside and undertake a tempting dish. If he should, he should not be discouraged because very frequently many efforts and much will power will have to be exerted. If he will just remember what great things and rewards are awaiting him from heaven, he will not yield to the hunger lust. Deu. 12:20, 21.

A common belief that one must remain indoors and perhaps in bed throughout a fast of any duration is entirely erroneous and is based on the assumption that we derive our strength and energy directly from the food that is consumed. A certain feeling of languor may be present during the early or latter days of a fast. A working man can continue working if his work is not overly strenuous. His prayer, however, would not be as concentrated and effective.

Before arising in the morning, one should exercise gently in bed and breathe deeply. This will counteract any dizziness and any other strange feelings that may occur at first. Plenty of water should be taken; this should be taken slowly.

HOW TO FAST

Usually these symptoms are only felt during the first few days and disappear entirely later on (When hunger returns the weakness experienced will be real). Never rise from any position suddenly. The purpose of this is to get the blood in circulation so you won't experience fainting.

After the body toxins have been consumed, eliminated. and oxidized, one will feel stronger mentally and physically. Pains, dizziness, weakness and peculiar feelings will have disappeared; all of the various organs and parts of the body, as well as the sense faculties, will be revitalized. Spiritually, one will feel as if the demons in hell are turned against him. The trials encountered at this time are numerous; naturally, the Devil doesn't want to see a child of God make headway toward FAITH. It simply means defeat for Satan. Jesus' greatest testing was after He had fasted forty days and forty nights. BEFORE HE PERFORMED A MIRACLE, HE FASTED. FASTING AND PRAYER DRIVES OUT ALL UNBELIEF AND DOUBT. Luke 4, Psalm 109:22-31 and Psalm 35:13.

It is doubtful if you will ever have such trials as the strange ones that come up while fasting or at the close of the fasting and praying period. To succeed SPIRITUALLY WITH GOD, IT IS ABSOLUTELY NECESSARY TO PRAY WHILE FASTING AND TO PRAY FERVENTLY. Here is the result: THERE IS NO SUCH GRAND, GLORIOUS, AND WONDERFUL EXPERIENCE IN ALL THE WORLD AS THE MARVELOUS ONE BROUGHT BY PRAYING AND FASTING. WORDS CANNOT DESCRIBE THE BLESSINGS THAT THIS WILL BRING ABOUT. PRAYERS THAT YOU HAVE BEEN PRAYING FOR YEARS WILL BE ANSWERED. YOUR DISEASES OR THE SICKNESS OF OTHERS THAT YOU WILL HAVE BEEN PRAYING ABOUT WILL PISAPPEAR. Your loved ones will be saved. You will have power and answers to prayer that you never realized was possible before.

Although various complications, many of which have been enumerated, appear while fasting, such as fainting, fever, dizziness, headaches, a tendency to vomit, severe sharp pains in the abdomen, weak knees, short breath, sleeplessness, or sleepiness all of the time, nervousness, vexation, foul breath, watery nose, sneezing, backache, burning kidneys, sideache, etc., THESE DO NOT ALL APPEAR AT ONCE, PERHAPS ONLY ONE OR TWO may be noticed by one individual in the entire fast. Please do not be alarmed, as this is just a natural result from the fast and in nearly all cases is only experienced during the first part of the fast. Usually hot water drinking, enemas and exercise will stop the condition. After the body is cleansed the condition will subside. Many times pains in abdomen are caused by drinking cold water too fast. The change to hot water will remedy the condition. The "Oxydation" of the "Waste" material causes the FEVER. Large enemas whenever necessary are helpful.

HOW LONG SHOULD WE FAST?

Until we definitely know that God has heard our prayer so we can acquire "THE POWER" that Jesus speaks of, to do the seemingly "impossible." We should fast and pray then regardless of whether or not this requires one meal, seven days or a complete fast of several weeks, forty days or until true hunger returns, which is a long fast. We can have a fast—through victorious experience.

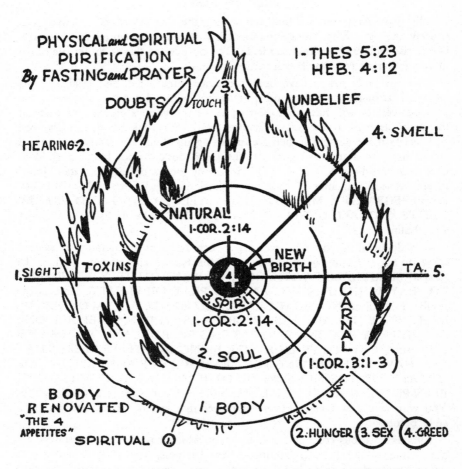

CHART No. IX. The BONFIRE, MAN ANALYZED AND DIAGRAMMED

The vital energies are freed from the laborious task of digesting, converting, and pushing food material through thirty feet of tubing, not to speak of the energy required for increased rapidity of heart action. Just as soon as all of this energy is released by the abstention of food, OXYDATION BEGINS WITHIN THE BODY, which IS NOTHING MORE THAN A BONFIRE IN WHICH ALL OF THE WASTE POISONS ARE CONSUMED.

The (1) body, (2) soul, (3) spirit, and (4) NEW BIRTH are depicted together with his five sense faculties of (1) sight, (2) hearing, (3) touch, (4) smell, and (5) taste. It is pleasing these sense faculties that lead to the gratification of the four appetites (see bottom of chart) that prevent the child of God from obtaining the better things. The natural appetites are larger than the spiritual appetite, but turn to the "Wells of Living Water Chart," after the fast and the appetites are reversed. (Faith ignores our sense evidence).

Chapter IX

FASTING IN RELATION TO THE PHYSICAL BODY

Is fasting harmful to the physical body? This question has been raised more than any other question concerning the subject The study of fasting, in the light of modern medical science cannot be harmful in the least. Fasting purifies and cleanses the body; it permits a balancing of the circulation absolutely essential to good health; it allows the various eliminating organs to dispose of the effete material in the system, and to oxidize or burn up the useless matter which has accumulated in the body, like ashes in the grate.

When a fast is begun, the first things which are oxidized and eliminated by the body are those useless materials floating about within it in the form of mal-assimilated food material, which sometimes choke the small blood vessels and congest the lymph vessels. In other words, THE VERY THINGS WHICH WE WISH TO ELIMINATE FROM THE SYSTEM ARE THOSE WHICH NATURE ACTUALLY DISPOSES OF FIRST OF ALL. Fasting is house-cleaning to the body. The Holy Spirit, then, is given a clean temple to dwell in. Cleanliness is also GODLINESS. When assimilation stops, the processes of elimination are greatly accelerated. We will show four methods used in this process.

THE FOUR MEANS TO HOUSE CLEANING

(1) The SKIN, by way of the pores, is one channel by which much toxic wastes are eliminated. Far more wastes are removed through our pores during a fast than at any other time. This is one reason Jesus said, "wash your face." It is also a good practice to bathe frequently.

(2) The KIDNEYS: This is why much water drinking is so highly beneficial. It dilutes the urine which constantly washes out the poisons that are poured into the kidneys.

(3) The LUNGS play an important part in this house cleaning process. It would seem almost unbelievable that loads of poison are exhaled in the fast through the nostrils from the oxygenation of the blood. The same amount of poison is released through the nostrils and lungs as through the kidneys, bowels and skin. All persons smell alike during the first part of the fast and a person familiar with fasting will recognize that the odor is that of a brother or sister, fasting, and should rejoice in his or her heart that his brother or sister is fulfilling some of the works of the Lord rather than criticize. If a person is praying and fasting the way he should, it should not bother him. If you don't want to have obnoxious breath around your neighbor, get some menthol crystals at the drug store. A very fine crystal particle will dissolve on the tip of your tongue so that your breath will not be noticed for a long time; there will be such a small amount in the tiny crystal that it will never be able to get back of your tongue far enough to get into the stomach. The

reason that I have mentioned this point, is that some folk have chewed gum when fasting and the amount of sugar in the gum would be almost enough to break the fast. The menthol crystal will be stronger than gum, more lasting in the berath and will be too small to reach the stomach. This is only a suggestion. Bad breath is a sign that the house cleaning process is going on. This vapor that comes from the lungs will clear up later on in the fast and the breath, as well as the taste in the mouth will become as CLEAN AND ODORLESS as that of a baby, believe it or not.

(4) The BOWELS are the fourth channel of elimination; it would be good if they would move every day or two but often they move with less frequency while on the fast, and do not be alarmed. Take large enemas if necessary; elevate the bag high.

Since all four of these methods of elimination are at work, is it any wonder then, that fasting is a way towards health? Even when one is in good health fasting prevents disease.

Fasting is the most powerful and the quickest agent known to cure functional ailments. Especially is this true of stomach disorders. In a long fast, a new-like stomach is acquired. That is why it is very necessary to break the fast carefully with fruit juices, followed by fresh fruit for several days.

If a person is in an adverse state of health, his eyes, throat, liver, glands, blood and even the kidneys a little later, become REJUVENATED and greatly benefitted. This is a natural law of God and this physical side is touched upon so that we will realize that fasting and prayer to God is harmless to the body. It would be unreasonable to think that Christ would ask us to fast if it would hurt us physically. We have a good God, and He asks us to do nothing that will hurt or harm us. One can FAST a long period of time and secure GREAT SPIRITUAL RESULTS WITHOUT BODILY HARM, and in addition, receive physical benefit.

If one is afraid that he is harming himself in fasting, and fearful, that person cannot obtain spiritual results from the fast. The Lord certainly does not want us to come to him in fear, so that is absolutely one thing that has to be dismissed from the mind entirely.

IS FASTING STARVATION?

Absolutely not! Fasting and starvation are two different things. To illustrate: The complete fast begins from the time you leave off one meal, and it ends after a large part of the body weight is lost, usually when true hunger returns (Matt. 4:1-4). It may last several weeks and longer. Jesus' fast lasted forty days before true hunger returned. In His fast, he fasted naturally, just like you or I would. When a man has a KEEN APPETITE, and is *hungry* at the end of a long FAST, like Jesus, it is an indication of good health. Any physician will tell you that a man with a good appetite is in good health.

At the end of a complete fast hunger sets in; at this point starvation begins if the fast is continued after true hunger returns. It was when starvation had just begun, at the end of Jesus' fast, when the devil sought to take advantage of Jesus by tempting Him. Satan dislikes to see God's children fast with prayer, because it means his quicker defeat. Fasting is like "dynamiting" Satan.

Starvation begins after most of the body weight is lost. It usually begins after true hunger returns which is hardly ever before twenty-one days, and may last longer than forty or sixty days. It is difficult to state the exact time when starvation sets in. It varies with different individuals. Fat people can fast much longer than thin ones.

The end of starvation is death. Death occurs after an individual has continued a fast after true hunger has returned and usually long after starvation sets in. Some confusion exists here. When you hear that someone died of starvation in a sea-wrecked vessel in two or three days, there is some mistake. A person can easily get cold or become frightened to death in a few hours time, or a few days time, more or less, but never starves to death in that short period if he has good water to drink. He could also worry to death in as short a time.

A human being is like a vital electric plant that is so constructed that ordinarily it is supplied with power from the dynamo, but may run for a considerable length of time on the battery current, for each of the millions of cells of the body is a cell similar to the most perfect cell of a storage battery. Fasting stops the dynamo and automatically turns the switch to the battery current, which is just as capable of sustaining life as the current from the dynamo. The capable physical individual has more capacity than one with a weak constitution.

In Yeo's PHYSIOLOGY, we find the longest case on record. "The patient, suffering from a gunshot wound in the abdomen, lived four months without any food. His weight decreased from 159 to 60 pounds. Every function was almost dormant, thought was unimpaired, the brain was unusually clear" (this is always the case of anyone who is fasting) "and the brain was found to have suffered no loss in size." The percentage of decrease of different parts of the organism in this fast, as well as others considered, is given by Mr. Yeo:

FAT	97%	BLOOD	17%
SPLEEN	63%	LIVER	56%
MUSCLE	30%	NERVE CENTERS	0%

A human being cannot starve to death in several weeks of fasting if he has water. One can die if he has worries or becomes frightened, either with food and drink, or without food and drink. One cannot drink milk or coffee when fasting, to do so is dieting and not fasting. Nothing at all is to be drunk except water. It is a purifying agent, and is necessary to wash out the poisons in the system.

Unless one's work is unusually heavy, and he is not continually praying, it is not necessary to give up his job. If he is not getting sufficient exercise in praying or work, he should take exercise regularly to assist the fast. Then it is eaiser to fast and very beneficial as well; the weakness leaves more readily and the fast gets underway much quicker. The exercise keeps the blood circulating. However, if we pray as we should, one will get all of the action and exercise that is needed, because real praying is hard work and this is what we want if we are to see great spiritual results. Of course, one's rest and sleep should be carried out as usual. If possible, have more rest when fasting than when not fasting. More rest may be required, although one does not seem to miss sleep like he would while eating.

THE BIBLE IS AHEAD OF SCIENCE

The "blood," or "life" of the flesh is the last part of the body to be consumed in the fast after starvation sets in. This is when the fast is carried into starvation.

Credit is given William Harvey for a great medical discovery in 1615 A.D. "The circulation of blood. Life is blood or the circulation of blood." This is supposed to be a great milestone in the history of medical science, but if you check into the Holy Scriptures, one finds that this is not a new discovery at all. Thousands of years before William Harvey's day, God told Moses this very same thing, Lev. 17:11. "For the life of the flesh is in the Blood." (Also Gen. 9:4 and Deut. 12:23) If the Bible was studied along with science, the scientists of the day would not make so many changes and errors and would be more up to date.

THE BLOOD AT WORK

I shall explain a little more about the cleansing process that is brought about by the blood. The blood, as you know, is driven by the heart, through the arteries, into the capillaries, which nourish and strengthen the body. It then returns, by means of the capillaries by another route, the veins, to the heart from whence it is drawn to the lungs.

The blood starts on its arterial journey, bright red and rich, laden with life-giving properties. It returns by the venous route, poor, blue and dull, being laden down with waste matter of the system. It goes out like a fresh stream from the mountains; it returns as a stream of sewer water. In a fast, the stream is far more polluted than when not fasting. This foul stream goes to the right auricle of the heart. When this auricle becomes filled, it contracts, and forces the stream of blood through an opening in the right ventricle of the heart, which in turn sends it on to the lungs, where it is distributed by millions of hair-like blood vessels to the air cells of the lungs .

The foul stream of blood is now distributed among the millions of tiny air cells in the lungs. Air is inhaled and the oxygen comes into contact with the impure blood through the thin walls of hair-like blood vessels of the lungs, walls thick enough to hold the blood, but thin enough to admit oxygen. When the oxygen comes in contact with the blood, a form of combustion takes place, and the blood takes up oxygen and releases carbonic acid gas, generated from the waste products and poisonous matter which have been gathered up by the blood from all parts of the system. The blood thus purified and oxygenated is carried back to the heart again, rich, red and bright, and laden with life-giving properties and qualities. Upon reaching the left auricle of the heart, it is forced into the left ventricle, from whence it is again forced through the

52

arteries on its mission of life to all parts of the system. It is estimated that in a single day of twenty-four hours, 35,000 pints of blood traverse the capillaries of the lungs, the blood corpuscles passing in single file and being exposed to the oxygen of the air on both of their services.

If the air cells of the lungs were spread out over an unbroken surface, they would cover an area of fourteen thousand square feet. When one considers the minute details of the process alluded to, he is lost in wonder and admiration of our blessed Father's care and Omnipotence and Omniscience.

Considering the value that the lungs play in the cleansing of the blood, one should be interested in proper deep breathing and securing plenty of fresh air. More about this is found in author's booklet *"Because of Unbelief,"* see back cover. (This volume will show a person how to have tremendous Faith.)

First and foremost as the cause of disease is the congestion of blood containing morbid waste material of the organs and tissues of the body. This thickened blood, surcharged with products of imperfect metabolism, finds itself unable to pass freely through certain parts of the body, a necessary thing for perfect health. The damming up of certain organs and tissues produces an engorgement, which interferes with the free and natural functioning of that particular part .There are few of the disorders from which mankind suffers where this condition is not present, and it is no exaggeration to say that it is the principal cause of all disease.

The condition is brought about in the blood stream by the use of more food than the body actually requires for its repair and development. Food that is the excess food and the insufficient exercise of muscles to assimilate the nourishment prevents the complete utilization of the food. This requires a lot of unnecessary energy. Jesus calls it *"SURFEITING,"* Luke 21:34.

This is one of the contributing causes of skin blemishes, boils, growths such as cancers and turmors and diseases of the mucous membranes, such as tuberculosis, ovarian and womb disorders, and leucorrhea.

Consequently a cure depends upon the elimination of this congestion, and a readjustment of the habits governing eating, exercising, etc., so that the body may be freed from the encumbrances. The way to do this is by stopping the assimilation for a time by fasting. It is effective in producing quick results. The results are so astounding both physically and spiritually, that it is like a bird that has been in a cage being set free out in the wide open.

Man is so used to satiating himself to the utmost with the food at his immediate disposal, and gorging upon the fruits of conquest.

When nutritious food became plentiful the cravings of hunger became less, and the cultivation of epicurean appetites became more and more a vice. Man has actually suffered in a greater degree from this than from the forced hunger of scarcity and the struggle that is necessary to provide for food.

Occasionally through time some soul will cry out in protest against sensual gratifications, but the mad crowd has little heeded the words of our Master's voice and the teachings of the scriptures. They have not pursued the POWER of the spirit, but have made the belly their God and their bellies the graveyards of their souls.

The practice of temperance will come more abundantly to those who understand that the practice of good habits will bring about rapid physical and spiritual changes which will make for immediate happiness both now and tomorrow. Fasting will conserve tremendous energy that can be utilized in building up the temple of the Holy Spirit.

Other teachers besides the prophets and Christ, such as Krishna, Buddha, and Mohammed have even awakened the minds of their followers in some degree to the moral and ethereal desirability of control over sensual pleasures, the root of which is EATING.

WHAT MEDICAL MEN SAY

The earliest physicans were united in teaching that abstentious living was the key to good health. They advocated the denying of food to a diseased body.

Through the centuries thousands of teachers have come and gone with their circles of disciples who have practiced fasting for the cure of disease, but there are few that take the treatment seriously from their physicians. Possibly because it seems like an Utopian dream, too good to be true, or the regime to be followed is too strict and requires too much will power.

Some doctors, medical, and health authorities have publications that clarify this science of fasting, from the standpoint of health and the cure of disease. Some of these writers on the subject are: Dr. Tanner, Sinclair, Dr. McCoy, Dr. Shaw Haskell, Dr. Dewey, Bernarr Macfadden, Dr. Jno. Cowan, Tilden Brook, Dr. R. Walter, and others.

Dr. Frank McCoy in his book, "THE FAST WAY TO HEALTH," states: "I have made a most exhaustive study of every method of cure from mind cure to modern surgery and gland therapy, and I HAVE NEVER FOUND A SINGLE METHOD THAT COULD APPROACH EVEN CLOSELY, IN ITS RESULTS, THE BENEFITS WHICH COME FROM SOME FORM OF THE FASTING CURE." Some of these volumes can be secured from your library.

Dr. McCoy treats his patients by fasting and dieting methods. He also prescribes a very long fast for some conditions, for both sicknesses and disorders of women and men. Most of his book gives illustrations and examples of his patients placed on a fasting or dieting treatment. If more physicians would practice this method of healing there would be less sickness.

Fasting has a distinct value in obtaining and retaining PERFECT HEALTH. In early times, Avicenna, the great Arabian physician, quite clearly sensed the value of fasting, since he often prescribed as much as a three-weeks fast for his patients; especially for syphilis and smallpox. Dr. Isaac Jennings as early as 1822 employed fasting successfully as an aid in almost every kind of ailment which he treated.

Fasting has proven a divine aid to the body's own processes of self recovery. Fasting in ailments such as asthma, hay fever, constipation, headaches, colds, skin disorders, arthritis and rheumatism, blood diseases, and anything else along the line of the blood and functional diseases has proven almost a miracle in their recovery. Benefits have been observed in nervous and mental disorders, paralysis, semi-paralysis, neurasthenia, and in some forms of insanity. (Please bear in mind that we are talking about natural divine aids and not DIVINE HEALING in this section, except that by FASTING AND PRAYER THE LORD CAN HEAL US OF ANY SICKNESS REGARDLESS OF WHETHER

IT IS INCURABLE OR NOT. This would be divine healing. Many incurable diseases by man are demons. Demons cannot be cured. They are cast out. It often requires prayer and fasting to do so.

When food is withheld oxydation begins within the body, which is nothing more than a collection of refuse gathered for a bonfire, in which waste poisons are burnt up just as a person would gather up the trash in his yard and burn it up in his incinerator. THIS IS INDICATED SOMETIMES BY A FEVER WHICH SETS IN DURING THE EARLY STAGES OF THE FAST, AND BY HEADACHES AND OTHER SYMPTOMS. (Consult Chart No. IX, Man Analyzed and Diagrammed.)

FASTING DOES NOT REDUCE, BUT INCREASES ENERGY AND HEAT OF THE BODY by the combustion of the waste poisons by a process of oxydation, so that waste becomes the fuel for its own destruction and elimination from the body. The process of combustion becomes a source of added bodily heat for the faster's comfort, as well as a source of added energy and power for bringing about revitalization, cleansing, and restoration of health.

Fasting gives the body a much needed holiday, a vacation. It never occurs to one that the body seldom ever has a rest from its ordinary labors. We overtax and overload all the organs with by-products of our wrong living, eating, drinking and thinking. We do not grant these millions of little cells which labor so incessantly for our physical well-being a rest, no not even a SAB-BATICAL REST. Most folk would be far better off if they would pray and fast at least one day a week. They would be better physically and spiritually. Most early churches, especially the Methodists, had at least one fast day a week.

Fasting RETAINS THE YOUTHFUL COMPLEXION AND APPEAR-ANCE, FASTING DEFERS OLD AGE AND KEEPS THE BODY YOUNG. Old age is both a biological and mental abnormality. Where it results from accumulated impurities and deposits. Abstention from food will help to remove the accumulations and thus defer the physiological process incident to old age. We are only as old as the number of dead cells we have in our body. Fasting converts dead cells into food fuel. This explains why we look so much younger after fasting.

With the PHYSICAL HOUSECLEANING GOES A MENTAL HOUSE-CLEANING. I have personally seen pessimism, gloom, discouragement, anger, grudges, fear, morbidity, despondency, worry, fussiness, mental tensions, per-versions, vile and depraved thoughts, excitability, other forms of mental con-ditions, and bad habits disappear completely after the bodily purification is accomplished. Bodily purification leads to spiritual purification. Demons many times, feed on food filth and carnality; many times fasting unlooses them and makes a person free from demons and disease.

Even the HEALTH AUTHORITY, Bernarr Macfadden, tells us: "The body intimately influences the higher soul-powers during a fast, I definitely know. Physical renovation and purification lead to spiritual renovation and puri-fication. I have experienced a sublimation of the Spirit during a prolonged fast which is difficult to put into words. It must be experienced to be known. There is a spring to the step, a feeling of joyous release, of gladness which fairly overwhelms one. There is, too, an exaltation of spirit, a broad and more generous sympathy, love and understanding for all things and for all mankind, a feeling of well-being, and of peace with God, with one's fellowman, with the world, and with all things which are a part of our everyday living."

If this is the experience of a person interested in the physical welfare of individuals, how much greater would be the experience of those who would "SPECIALIZE," in POWER AND FAITH WITH GOD through FASTING AND PRAYER?

WHY DO I HAVE A HEADACHE WHEN FASTING

When a meal is eaten, one half of our blood immediately is drawn upon to take care of the food consumed; consequently, we feel weak immediately after a meal and should not do heavy, strenuous work at that time. Coaches instruct athletes not to eat heavy food before a game, or better yet, fast several meals preceding the game. If it is best from a scientific and physical standpoint to abstain from food so that more can be done on the athletic field of batttle, how much more important it is that man should work more effectively on God's battlefield, by prayer and fasting.

Although it may sound as strange as fiction, the fact that you have a headache is an indication that you need the fast. This is what happens: all of your blood is used to carry off the poison and toxins when you omit a meal, the blood stream becoming polluted with toxic material and excreted matter. As the circulation carries the blood through all parts of the body as we have shown, it enters the head, which causes it to ache. After the heaviest part of the housecleaning gets under way, usually after several days of fasting the headache gradually disappears and a feeling of more comfort than before fasting is felt. This is of course after the blood stream becomes purified by the fast. Many headaches are nothing more than caffeine headaches caused from coffee drinking. Fasting will remove these by consuming the caffeine.

If you eat a heavy meal, the blood would not have time to keep the system clean, so it goes to work where the food is, in the stomach, while the poisons, to some extent, continue in the body. This same reason will also explain why we feel weak during the first part of the fast and is why other symptoms sometimes appear while taking a protracted fast. The blood continues cleansing our bodies and the complexion clears and the skin takes on a healthy, rosy, natural, and normal color later on in the fast. Most participants will also become stronger physically day by day.

A certain Bible student fasted approximately two weeks. Before the fast the student made a muscle test by chinning himself eighteen times. On the ninth day of the fast, to show that fasting did no harm and did not weaken him later on, he was able to chin himself twenty-two times, or four times more than he was able to chin before taking the fast. The students were surprised, and moreover, these students on the campus, who had been eating three regular meals a day, were not able to chin as many times as the student who had fasted nine days. The writer was in the same Bible college when the contest took place, and can verify this.

Chapter X

THE PROPER CARE IN BREAKING THE FAST

It is very difficult to break the fast properly and very important. The importance of breaking the fast correctly and wisely cannot be over-emphasized. If you wish to avoid any consequences after your fast, please use plain common sense as well as heeding the following directions carefully. Very often an individual takes a fast of several weeks and gets along fine in the fast, but to his disappointment has uncomfortable physical difficulties while he is in the process of breaking the fast, which in practically all cases can be traced directly to his impatience to begin eating the accustomed rations days and weeks too soon.

If you have fasted very long, or have taken a complete fast, you have practically a brand new stomach and it will have to be adjusted to food again.

If you had your automobile engine overhauled, it would be necessary to break it in slowly for so many miles. If it were a major overhaul, you would have to run it at a lower R.P.M. even longer. The same thing applies to a new engine.

I had an airplane that had an 80 horsepower engine in it. I had it "majored" by an A. and E. mechanic. Before I could fly it, even at a low R.P.M., the motor was run, while on the ground, for about five hours. Then after it had been broken in sufficiently to fly, it was flown at low cruising speed for another five hours. These ten hours that were required to break in the engine, were broken down into short periods so the engine would be properly broken in safely.

Our bodies are the same way after a protracted fast. The longer the fast the more care it takes before resuming the regular diet again. Our stomach has to be broken in gradually and time is required between periods for rest, and for the gradual return of the assimilative functions of the body.

In the Bible days, Israel, the prophets and Christ were acquainted with the dietic laws of Moses, the prophets and Essenes, and knew about the hygiene necessary to break a fast, etc. But today most people are ignorant of this information. In a long fast the stomach is new, like a child's stomach. And when you break a fast, it must be done properly, so as not to injure the stomach. Any part of the body which is the temple of the Holy Spirit should not be injured.

After true hunger has returned, (in some instances, true hunger does not return) or if one finds it necessary and advisable to break fasting before hunger has returned, he should use only fresh citrus fruits. Oranges and grapefruits are the best to break it with, however, fresh tomato juice is very good. Grape juice from fresh grapes is very fine. Sauerkraut juice, if agreeable, is sometimes good for the second or third meal after the fast is broken. If the fast is seven days or under, it can be broken with whole fresh fruit for two or three meals and light soups the second day; the third day green vegetables and your regular diet from there on. Even a fast of two or three days will prevent one from sitting down at a table to eat a regular meal, if he wishes to feel comfortable after breaking the fast. But it is not so necessary to break this type fast as carefully as a fast that has been entered into for many days. (canned fruits are satisfactory when fresh fruits or juices are not available.)

If the fast is very long it will take several meals of fresh fruit juices, in small diluted quantities to correct natural tendencies. Your regular diet should not commence until at least an equal number of days, comparable to the number of days that you have fasted have elapsed. For instance, if you have fasted twenty-eight days, you should have a gradual breaking-in period of twenty-eight days before you take up a regular diet again. You should start out with your fruit juices for several days, your fresh fruit for two or three days more, then eat light soups, not too milky, for another two or three days, some green vegetables for another period. Gradually, little by little, break into the regular diet.

Since much weight is lost, the quickest way to gain that back is by drinking milk after several days of the above-mentioned schedule. Small amounts should be taken at first then larger and larger portions. CAUTION: Sometimes milk will cause the individual to bloat, and assimilation will be too great. If this should happen, or any other difficulty arises, it is because you are rushing the breaking-in period. The remedy is to eat less or cut out some of the food. If necessary, go back to fruit juices or fresh fruit again. If very severe, go back to FASTING and do not drink water. Take enemas often. This is a safe rule to follow, if any complication should develop while in the "breaking-in period.'

We urge you, by all means, to obtain our Book, "GLORIFIED FASTING." We feel this volume will give you more information on breaking the fast than any other volume available. We feel that every person who fasts much, should have it. It is called the "ABC of FASTING." 40 illustrations.

NOTICE: *THIS IS VERY IMPORTANT*

Do not rush your stomach. The longer you wait to regain your weight, the slower you start getting back to your regular eating, the better your physical condition will be afterward. If you fail to wait long enough, you will undo much that has been accomplished physically.

To eat a full meal during the conclusion of a protracted fast or even during the breaking-in period will shock the nervous system severely. Sometimes a nervous collapse, if not a complete nervous breakdown will be the result. THE PROPER BREAKING-IN PERIOD CANNOT BE OVER-EMPHASIZED TO THE FASTING CANDIDATE IF HE IS NOT TO SUFFER ANY AFTER EFFECTS. YOUR STOMACH IS TOO WEAK, FOR A LONG TIME, to handle the usual supply of food that it has been accustomed to digesting. Considering the large amount of weight that has been lost, it would overwork the stomach to restore this weight too soon, as the processes of digestion and assimilation require a great amount of nervous energy as well. Please do not worry about the weight that was lost or the slowness of your stomach and nervous energy to become adapted to normalcy, because your stomach will eventually become a stronger stomach and its functions will be restored to greater efficiency and your weight needed will be completely restored to normal. Even thin folk will gain more weight than they weighed before if they break the fast right.

It may require months of patience before all functions and the complete weight of an individual who has fasted forty days are completely restored. This does not mean that he will not feel good and will fail to have the great SPIRITUAL RESULTS that he sought. Plenty of rest and sleep should be had at this time.

PATIENCE is one of the fruits that will be developed by the fast. "FAITH WORKETH PATIENCE," One of the greatest things that is desired by the candidate is FAITH, as that is what is promised to us so that "NOTHING SHALL BE IMPOSSIBLE UNTO YOU." The patience that it takes to fast and to break the fast, the great will power continually being developed in us, all go towards opening up the treasure house of heaven for our welfare.

Meat and heavy food should not be eaten until about the same number of days have elapsed that the candidate has fasted; even then one really does not require so much food and since your stomach is actually smaller (more normal) you really do not care for such large amounts of food after the breaking-in period. Great will power will have to be used to avoid over-eating before the breaking-in period has expired. In fact, it may require more effort to break the fast properly than it did during the first few days that seemed so difficult to get started on the fast before hunger left. One must continually fight against over-eating and muster up all will power to do this. Even if one does not feel ill from improper eating one may lose certain physical results that would have stayed after the breaking-in period. A person should never go back to eating the foods that do not make a balanced, healthful, wholesome diet and foods that are deficient in the minerals and elements that the body requires. He should never give way to over-indulgences and excess again. The scriptures tell us to "be temperate in all things," Also "Feed me with food conveniently for me."

The loss of weight in a fast is about one pound a day. This, of course, depending upon the weight of a person before fasting. A very heavy person will lose more than a pound a day, while a thin person will sometimes lose less than this after the first few days of the fast. During the first few days as much as two or more pounds will be lost daily. This is due mostly to the fact that waste material is quickly breaking down and is being eliminated. It has been estimated that Christ lost approximately thirty-seven to forty pounds. Toward the end of fasting, one will lose slightly less each day. Much more weight is lost when working heavily.

The weight that is lost is gained back after the normal routine of eating is undertaken, following the breaking of the fast. If a person was overweight before fasting, a few weeks after the fast he will be more nearly normal in weight, and if he continues to eat moderately, the person will remain at almost normal weight. If the person was thin before fasting (and thin people, too, should fast and pray), he will put on weight after he begins to eat regularly again. In other words, protracted fasting normalizes the weight. Fasting also normalizes practically all functions of the human body and this is a law of nature which is a law of God. Fasting is the greatest and quickest curative agent known to man. Because fasting seems unpopular to many, and unreasonable, is no reason why anyone has a right to condemn it. ONLY NARROW-MINDED PEOPLE CONDEMN SOMETHING THEY KNOW NOTHING ABOUT. Nobody has a right to condemn anything that they know nothing of. In the former days people were not ignorant of this great health measure, but today it seems lost to many. (Search the Bible.)

The "ABC" of FASTING gives a complete day by day menu for breaking any length of FAST. Forty illustrations show you details. Order from author. See last page.

Here is another testimony of a sister who fasted fourteen days.

On the 31st of December, 1945, my husband and I started on a consecration fast. We ate nothing during the entire fast; we did drink water. My husband fasted fourteen and I fasted nineteen days. My husband was delivered of the smoking habit and received the glorious Baptism of the Spirit. He was also very nervous, but was nervous no longer after the fast. I never was hungry on my fast. On the seventh day the Lord refilled me with power. We both attended services every day. We both felt better than we ever felt and had no weakness or headaches, except my husband who had a little at first. I thank Jesus for many who have begun to fast under "Hall."

I know that if you fast and pray you will be drawn closer to God. It is easier to testify and worship God. It is also one of the best ways to regain your health. You can feel the results as you continue day by day.

Grace Wilson
4010 Euclid Avenue,
San Diego 5, Calif.

AFRICAN FASTS FORTY DAYS

Dear Brother Hall:

I hope you would desire to notice that the Lord has enabled me to complete forty days and forty nights of fasting praying for a revival. During this forty day period, I saw Jesus standing at the foot of my bed many times. I feel like I have had a heavenly experience. I received many strange and glorious experiences. Some of the experiences were like Daniels. Since I am in the beginning of the breaking in period, I will have much to tell later on. May the Lord continue to bless you in your good work. Many are being stirred here.

With all my love, I am yours in Christ,
Peter Ashon
Obiara—MPEH
"Camp" Via Diaccove
Gold Coast West Africa

Chapter XI

THINGS FORBIDDEN TO EAT

In Genesis 2:9, 17, we have the creative act described, reading as follows: "Out of the ground made the Lord God to grow every tree that is pleasant to the sight and good for food; the tree of life also in the midst of the garden, and the tree of knowledge of good and evil." Verse seventeen: "But of the tree of the KNOWLEDGE OF GOOD AND EVIL, THOU SHALT NOT EAT OF IT: FOR IN THE DAY THAT THOU EATEST THEREOF THOU SHALT SURELY DIE."

The day soon drew near when Eve and Adam partook of food from a tree that was forbidden by God to enjoy. When one crosses the barrier of the will of God, whether it is eating, business or pleasure he is certain to reap the consequences. Spiritual and physical indigestion was the result of that dinner that contaminated the systems of Adam and Eve. It is lamentable that improper eating was one of the first causes of judgment. Man became the sickest of all creatures on the face of the earth. Disobedience and the giving way to our appetites to the wrong type of food forced God to change the diet of man, and man was thus forbidden to eat the HEALTH FOODS that were in the Garden of Eden. The food from the TREE OF LIFE which was the ideal food to give health and LIFE to man so that he could live on forever without dying, was also denied him.

These foods were just what the physical man should have always had. They would have kept him from sickness, weariness, and other such grievous things that would rapidly increase the tempo of death.

The diet of man was drastically changed. The "TREE OF LIFE" was no longer within the reach of man. Man now was suffered to eat his WAY BACK TO EARTH and that is what all people are doing today. Every bite of food that is eaten is just one more step closer to the grave. Every day is just one day nearer the end of time for man. The food that is eaten lacks something, no matter how "vitamized," or "mineralized," or how wholesome, is still short of a certain something that should produce the healing, health and physical life qualities of man forever. We must recognize this fact, for whether we like it or not, everyone of us are eating our way back into the ground, and the more we eat, the quicker we will "return unto the earth."

We find in Genesis 3:17-19: "Cursed is the ground for thy sake; IN SORROW SHALT THOU EAT OF IT ALL THE DAYS OF THY LIFE. (V. 19) IN THE SWEAT OF THY FACE SHALT THOU EAT BREAD; TILL THOU RETURN UNTO THE GROUND; for out of it wast thou taken: for dust thou art, and UNTO DUST THOU SHALT RETURN." How can one be healthy and live forever in the physical body while eating something that is cursed and "in sorrow eat of it all the days of our life." A great many

61

folk seem to be so taken up with the cares of this world and the cares of eating that it would seem they were planning to live on this planet without Christ forever.

An individual can discontinue the practice of eating and avoid that which is "CURSED" BY GOING ON A "HUNGER STRIKE." The only thing that is taken is that which is not cursed, "WATER," FRESH AIR, AND REST. Carnality that is caused by food leaves in several days and the weakness that one has, which is caused by food contamination, leaves in a few days more. Is it any wonder then that the individual seems to be in another world. There is no great curse to curse his body, to even hinder him in the slightest way as far as his corruptible appetites are concerned from contacting God and developing a high spiritual standard of faith.

The individual at this point is like Adam and Eve were after the fall, before starting out on the regime of eating of the ground all the days of their life in "SORROW."

As this individual continues the fast indefinitely, he will find that he is getting along nicely in the fast whether it be twenty-one, twenty-eight, or forty days.

At this point he notices that his weight is falling approximately one pound per day. Of course this should not continue too long. There is something that is necessary to prevent it. This is not, contrary to public opinion, "FOOD" in the sense of the word that we know food now, because this food as we have shown is cursed and makes man cursed physically. It brings him right back to the earth.

What is this element or substance that he needs to continue without going back to dust? Man cannot go back to eating very easily at this stage. He has done without it too long.

The answer to this question is found in the paradise of the new city of Heaven that descends out of heaven that has, "THE TREE OF LIFE." This tree bears twelve manner of fruits and yields her fruit every month: The leaves of the tree are for the healing of the nations. And there shall be "NO MORE CURSE." Rev. 22:2-3.

He cannot partake of the tree of life yet, and he cannot get what the body has to have; to his sorrow he must go back and see if he can break into eating again and this will be a slow process because a meal at this time would not be received at all by the stomach. It could not be digested, and would nearly wreck the individual, if not *kill he* who made the attempt. A breaking-in period on fresh fruit juices and fresh fruit is *absolutely necessary* before regular eating is resumed. Your attention is called to the chapter, "THE PROPER CARE IN BREAKING THE FAST." It is important that this be studied carefully.

Before this breaking-in period, and before he is able to eat his accustomed meals, the Christian would be like Adam and Eve were immediately after they were driven from the Garden and were forced to start eating food similar to the food we get today.

Most diseases, as I have again and again pointed out in my lectures, are nothing more than a pollution of the blood-stream and cellular tissues through the introduction, development, and accumulation of toxins, ferments, waste, debris, or other poisonous matter within the physical system. To an extent, the ordinary functional processes of self-elimination cannot handle them in the normal and regular way of excretion. Over-eating of foods not needed by the system, which remain as poisonous ferments in the colon; vitiating the blood and saturating the tissues and cells with poisons introduced into the body through impure air, tobacco-poisoning, drug medicines, drinking excessively of tea, coffee, colas, chocolate, cocoa, or aclholic beverages, refined sugar, white flour, and other processed and devitalized foodstuffs, condiments, spices, pepper, sauces, and other acid-forming agents, clog the system.

BLESSING OUR FOOD

If our bodies are the Temple of the Holy Spirit, by the reason of containing a soul, "This soul having been vitalized by the Holy Spirit," why should we have the right to defile it by over-indulgence, or by eating anything that is contrary to the Divine Dietician's Laws? How can we contaminate it by the use of alcohol, nicotine, or narcotics? These things not only abuse, but actually kill the physical body of man. These are part of the excesses spoken of in I Cor. 3:16, 17.

The purpose and place of eating should also be taken into consideration. In Ex. 23:25 we have a condition, that if exercised, brings a blessing. ("Ye shall bless thy God in service.) (Ye shall serve the Lord your God and he shall bless thy bread and thy water and will take sickness away from the midst of thee.)

The food that we eat is what makes us sick and die prematurely.

In Ex. 23:25, it sounds as though good health comes from a proper understanding of the word, as well as a proper understanding of the place that food has. If the proper food is blessed, we either with understanding of diet become sick, or with such food overcome sickness and gain health and strength. We can be assured that God will help our infirmities and take our sicknesses away. He states in Ex. 15:26: "I am the Lord that healeth thee." Read: Deut. 28th chapter; Lev. 17:10-14 with Lev. 11 and Lev. 19:26; Deut. 12:23; Deut. 13:23 and 5:9 with I Cor. 11:28-30.

Because of the great lack of thanksgiving at the table and the lack of prayer in our homes, we must learn the hard way, with sickness and suffering in our bodies. It would pay any household to take time to thank God, in a moment of prayer, for the food that He gives the people. It would also pay every person to heed the warning given in Phil. 3:19: "Whose end is DESTRUCTION, whose GOD is their BELLY and whose glory is their shame who mind earthly things."

There are literally thousands and thousands of God's people that are suffering from nothing more than auto-intoxication, and the sad thing is, they do not know it. They do not realize that by cutting down their food consumption, taking out such foods that are not helpful to the body, they could restore health, vigor, vitality, and healing. More spiritual power would also develop.

Medical men well know the potence and stimulating character of food. A doctor is called to the home of a sick person, his diagnosis in nearly all cases starts with the stomach. The very first thing he does is to look at the tongue. If your tongue is coated with white covering, you have indigestion. If your tongue is rather brown, you will find constipation, etc. The doctor then proceeds from there with his diagnosis, gives the prescription or remedy that in most cases will correct the faulty condition. It may be recognized here that much of our modern-day stomach disorders are the result of improper eating, assimilation, and elimination.

A Christian brother in a Southeastern Kansas town was suffering seriously with ulcers. He attended the divine healing services conducted by Dr. P. C. Nelson, now gone on to be with the Lord, a Baptist evangelist. In these services thousands of people had been anointed with oil and prayed for, according to James 5. Many were being healed. This brother being prayed for was healed. The following night in the service, this person rose to his feet and said: "I thank God for healing my body. I feel perfect tonight. For dinner I ate twelve large roasting ears of corn, a large steak, vegetables, ice cream and cake. Eating all of this did not seem to affect me in the least."

The Lord graciously healed this person, although he did not deserve it. Through ignorance, he had overlooked all of God's dietetical laws and had made his stomach God. I am very sorry to say, after a year from that date of healing, this man died and went on, we hope, to be with the Lord.

This person was completely healed at the time prayer was offered in his regard, but through his over-eating, as we have related, soon accomplished in reverse all that God had done for him.

Medical statistics reveal that 95% of the American people over eat and are auto intoxicated from food.

Over-eating is one of the greatest curses of our modern day. Before the machine age, man worked hard and long for the money he earned. He laboured, earning his bread by the sweat of his brow. Modern man does not. It is understandable that the men of the other age needed greater quantities of food to sustain their body.

Today men forget the fact that many of us are not in need of three large meals per day. Although many are of the opinion that unless a person eats three big meals a day he is being under-fed.

It is logical to believe that when a person is eating three to five meals a day, there is excess energy, and only a small amount of his energy is being used.

Today, the new age is in the making, and many of us fail to realize that while this change is being made, we are continuing in our old paths as far as food consumption is concerned. We should not only recognize the change in environment, but also in the life and work of modern man. We can be assured that many modern men and women would get along much better with only two, rather than three LARGE meals per day.

To those who are auto-intoxicated and really are in no need of the amount of food they are accustomed to eating, let them try this simple experiment: "Eliminate any one of your meals and to your great surprise you will be feeling much better than you had ever expected." If you are successful in eliminating one meal a day for thirty days, and feel that it has beneficial qualities, you will notice that at the end of this time you will continue this practice, fasting a meal per day. (That is, of course, unless one is not already under-fed.)

If you will continue the practice of fasting one meal per day, associating your fast with prayer, you will find new spiritual powers open to you. TRY IT, AND SEE THE RESULTS. I am sure you will be surprised!

LUST HUNGER

We can be assured that God hates the glutton, for in Psalms 78:29-34: "So they did eat, and were well filled: for he gave them their own desire."

"They were not estranged from their lust, But while their meat was yet in their mouths, the wrath of God came upon them, and slew the fattest of them, and smote down the chosen men of Israel," etc.

To eat when one does not actually need food is a double sin, "the sin of waste," and a sin against the body, bringing weakness and a short life.

It is too easily forgotten that it was Adam and Eve that also lusted after a new kind of food, "a food highly forbidden;" but not heeding the example, they ate and were required to suffer death through the sin of disobeying God.

The same thing is forgotten today, and when one would preach and expose these sins, too many will object.

"And they tempted God in their heart by asking meat for their lust, yea, they spake against God; they said, Can God furnish a table in the wilderness?"

God at first did not give them food readily here, they actually did not need it. This food was wanted to satisfy an appetite of LUST which is habit hunger.

God did, however give them "angel's food" and "sent them meat to the full. He gave them their own desire." And they were destroyed.

*A close study of the scriptures will show us clearly that sin is sin. The partaking of an over-amount of food is classed in the category of sin, because the same damage is done to the body, as that of alcohol, tobacco, dope etc.

This fact is also emphasized by Jesus Christ when he was tempted by Satan for forty days. He was commanded or requested to make the stones to become food. Jesus' answer was very efficient. "MAN SHALL NOT LIVE BY BREAD ALONE, BUT BY EVERY WORD THAT PROCEEDETH OUT OF THE MOUTH OF GOD." See Deut. 8:3 and Matt. 4:4.

Again Jesus shows what value the world will place on food when "The Son of man cometh. For as in the days that were before the flood, they were EATING AND DRINKING. So shall also the coming of the Son of man be."

Jesus is not critizing the eating to live. But He is greatly condemning the "living to eat," this is so prevalent everywhere. It is a sign of the last days. The sign that tells us of the soon coming of our Lord.
Matt. 24:37, 38. Eating is placed ahead of drinking. Many times "drink" in the scriptures means alcoholic or food drinks.

Adam and Eve were still on talking terms with God after they had partaken of the fruit of the tree of "knowledge of good and evil" before they were cast out of the "Garden of Eden" and were compelled to change their

---

*Brother Ted Fitch's books, *"OUR AFFLICTTIONS"* and *"PERFECT HEALTH,"* go into this subject very thoroughly (price .75 each). Address Ted Fitch, Council Bluffs. Ia. Brother Fitch's books give helpful diets and menus for Christians.

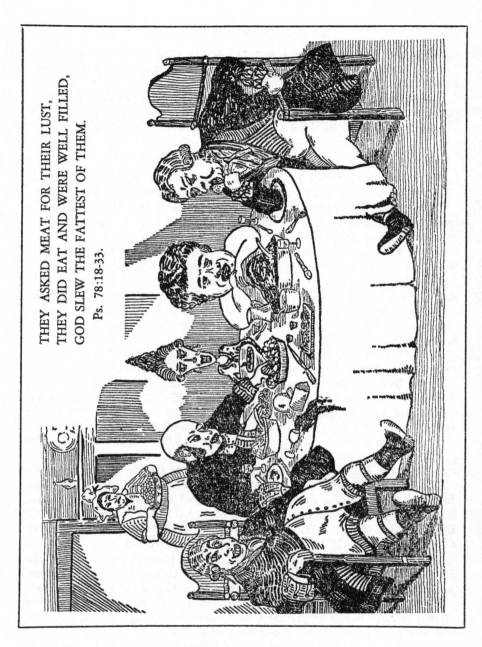

THEY ASKED MEAT FOR THEIR LUST,
THEY DID EAT AND WERE WELL FILLED,
GOD SLEW THE FATTEST OF THEM.
Ps. 78:18-33.

No. X THE GLUTTONS

The love of eating is the second root of all evil. It is definitely pointed out by Christ to be a last day sign. Matt. 24:38; Lk. 21:34. There is nothing wrong with the enjoyment of "eating to live," but it is wrong to just "LIVE TO EAT." There is a big difference. Ps. 78:33 shows us plainly that this is the cause of sickness. More were destroyed from gluttony than alcoholism.

diet from that of the luscious garden fruit to that which was cursed. But they had to consume large quantities to secure the small amounts of nourishment. Their position before the new diet began, which was to be a diet similar to the food that we now eat, would be comparable to one who had been on a long fast, before he started to break it. He, too, no doubt, would have come close enough to the Lord to be on talking terms with Him.

Since the ground and food were now cursed, it undoubtedly took awhile for Adam and Eve to become accustomed to this food; it was similar to a person breaking his fast, which would have to be broken gradually.

Medical science knows there is something lacking, something missing in the diet of man; this explains the reason that all kinds of prescriptions, remedies, and patent medicines are being tried. Everyone that has something wrong is trying everything imaginable to arrive at what seems to be the MISSING "LIFE" FOOD. Thank God, this will be found after "THE CURSE HAS BEEN REMOVED" (Rev. 22).

Divine healing is through one part of the atonement that Jesus paid for. This was to remove that part of the curse. It is actually Jesus' will for everyone to be healed because He paid the price, "with His stripes we are healed."

Chapter XII

RESULTS OF FASTING AND PRAYING

St. Paul has probably inspired more men and women to Jesus Christ than any other person. His teachings are more looked up to and sought for our welfare in the church today than any other writer. After Paul's conversion he began his career with a three-day fast, Acts 9:9. If every convert would follow Paul's example by fasting three days, meditating and praying after his conversion, there would be fewer backsliders and more chosen vessels in the Lord's service. According to Gal. 1:17, Paul then went to Arabia, "Neither went I up to Jerusalem to them which were apostles before me," preparation had to be made, Christ had to be woven into his theology. Changes had now to be made. A mystery is supposed to cover his stay in Arabia, but of the effect of fasting on a man of Paul's character, there remains no mystery. Since he says of his Christian career, he was "in fastings often" (II Cor. 11:27), there can be little doubt that he fasted in Arabia, when all circumstances make it very probably correct and were most favorable for a fast. The result was that he returned to Damascus and began to preach Christ in power and demonstration of the Spirit. He became a spiritual giant for God. All of us need to go into "THE WILDERNESS," or "INTO ARABIA" BEFORE BEGINNING TO PREACH CHRIST, or if there is that something lacking in your life, even if you have the Baptism of the Holy Spirit, the FASTING EXPERIENCE is also there for you. There would be success instead of so many failures in the ministry, the power and demonstration in the Spirit would be manifested and gifts of the Spirit would commence to operate. If there is any one agency that can do this quickly and perfectly, it is the consecration fast. This is the certain method to anointing.

We have been too busy with "much serving" as ministers and have missed the power for the highest service, because we have failed to follow Brother Paul in his fasting as he has invited us when he says: "Walk as ye have us for an example;" surely, since he was "in fasting often" this is included in the example. In II Cor. 11:23 St. Paul says: "Are they ministers of Christ? I am more"— largely because he was "in fastings often." All of the verse, II Cor. 11:27, reads: "In weariness and painfulness, in watchings often, IN HUNGER AND THIRST, IN FASTINGS OFTEN, in cold and nakedness," is herewith given to show that Paul distinguishes the doing without water in his hunger from that of fasting which is doing without food only, but includes the drinking of water. Here is the secret of being more than a mere minister, in the sense of Paul. All who will take his words to heart can excel by using this glorious agency.

This is for all believers as well as ministers like Paul. "Be followers of me, as ye have us for an example," Phil. 3:17, is evident from the manner in which he refers to fasting and prayer, I Cor. 7:5, "Defraud ye not one the other, except it be with consent for a time, that ye may give yourselves to fasting and prayer." These words cannot be construed as being addressed alone to ministers, although they are included. They are addressed to all and it is a routine work of salvation that needs to be worked out after we are converted. Verse six, "I speak this by permission, and not of commandment," pertains to the marriage relationship of the sex appetite which should be denied in fasting and later on after approximately three days in the fast the desire would have disappeared any way. If the married couple wish all the happiness there is in wedlock, before you ever argue with one another about breaking up, try the fast way and to your surprise things can be healed so that you will want to go on another honeymoon. Try it out and see, it is also an inexpensive method, a money saver!

In Acts 13:1, 2: "They ministered to the Lord and FASTED." The result was to finding the will of God. Paul and Barnabas were to be separated to the work whereunto God had called them. It seems the Holy Ghost hasn't a chance in the churches nowadays; but give the Holy Ghost a chance to lead by fasting and praying and see the results.

II Cor. 6:1-5: "We then approving ourselves as the ministers of God in much patience . . . in fastings." Surely, if he could not approve himself a minister of God without fasting, how can the rest of us presume to do so? Paul certainly was acquainted with the value of this tonic.

Ministers can be their own evangelist by a season of fasting and prayer and will do more good than a stranger could possibly do without it; there will be less psychology and stories, but more spiritual power and demonstration as well as fervor and zeal in the revival.

Bible students can obtain the choicest post-graduate course in the university of the Spirit by uniting for a season of prayer and fasting. They can become better commentators on the Pauline Epistles by obtaining the Pauline FER-VENCY and ZEAL than ever thought possible, by just following Paul's example.

Bible conferences, fellowship meetings, basket dinner gatherings in the church, feasting, jubilees, musical services, and prayer meetings are conducted. Why not have a fasting-prayer and consecration-fast anointing services and conferences? The results have been astounding in the places where they have been held, as we shall presently tell you.

Even Jesus, after He received the Holy Spirit did not begin to manifest His Sonship until after He had fasted forty days. All children of God in order to manifest will need to follow Jesus in fasting and prayer. There is no other way to have a complete manifestation but by fasting and prayer, and there is, according to St. Paul, no other remedy for the groaning and suffering of creation than a complete manifestation of the children of God, as far as is possible here on earth.

Rom. 8:19-22: "The whole creation groaneth and travaileth in pain togther until now, and waiteth for the manifestation of the Sons of God for the creature was made subject to vanity." Even the music of the birds is in a minor key, all animal life is groaning with unpleasant sound, there are sounds of discord, the wealing and wailing, barking and meowing, the howling and growling, all a sign of sin and pain, the noise on the street, the clanging of the wheels on the street car, the sound of your automobile, the howling and whistling of the wind in windy weather, all these and much more all go on to remind us of the groaning of the creation. Why? The answer to it is because the sons of God and more of the children of God are not MANIFESTING. The crying of countless millions in Europe, the cries of starving multitudes that are dying all over the world after this second world war have reached a high, shrill pitch of suffering. It is all because the sons of God are not manifesting themselves. The cripples, the sick, the suffering, the insane asylums filled with the distressed, and hospitals running over with the sick and wounded, the groanings of suffering humanity everywhere are because the sons of God do not have the vision on how to manifest. The Laodicean denominational bound Church have so many riches, comfortable pews, stained glass windows and the CHRIST who is supposed to be in HIS own church is left outside. Now He is knocking to a few individuals. Think of it, Jesus on the outside of His own church. The so-called Christians and makeshifts of Church and state are of no avail as a remedy and have actually become a reproach to Christ, and prolong the struggle and sufferings of millions. Under the sombre, laden skies a shaft of hope is revealed to us. In the providence of God there is only one remedy that will terminate the groaning instead of merely suppressing it as other agencies do, that remedy is the "manifestation of the sons of God." Our complete manifestation, of course, takes place when the Spirit quickens us when "The adoption, to wit, the redemption of our body" (Rom. 8:24), occurs, but we have an "earnest expectation" available now, not for just a few individuals among the sons of God but the entire body of them. One can be a child of God all his life without "MANIFESTING" in this sense. Yes, one can even receive the Baptism of the Holy Spirit and not fully manifest. On the day of Pentecost the one-hundred-twenty received the Baptism and the fire, backed by not only days of real prayer, but as they were in the upper room continually they had many days of FASTING. The result, the world's greatest revival. It shook the whole city and countryside. These women and men who were in the upper room began to MANIFEST AND SOMETHING HAPPENED. They were all in one accord and their unity knew neither divisions nor sectarianism.

FASTING CAUSES CHANGE IN ENVIRONMENT

Fish that are to be moved from one aquarium to another are put on a three-day fast before they are shipped. When they get to their destination they are eager to eat their food and the loss is insignificant. If the fish are fed immediately before the trip they nearly always refuse to eat the food while in transit and die en route.

Both fish and animals of all kinds, when placed in confinement or new environment when hungry, will take food in it, but if they are put into the confinement when not hungry, they will rebel against it and refuse to take food; futhermore they very often become sick.

When a change in environment is to take place, animals as well as men should go on a fast and it is much easier to become adapted to the changes. This is also true when undertaking a long journey, one's stomach does not become so easily upset if he fasts one or more meals before starting the trip. The environment of the Christian changes from the natural to the spiritual after the fast is undertaken. See CHART on THE CHANGE IN ENVIRONMENT.) This will illustrate to us, "WHY FAST." It is to secure the great Atomic Spiritual Results. God is a Spirit and we cannot come to Him to worship Him as we should without seeking Him in the Spirit. To do this we must also lose sight of the natural. Fasting and prayer is the answer.

In a fast, the senses diminish until the natural is placed in the background. Consciousness becomes affected so that it is focused on the new environment. The environment sense of the fishes was dulled by three days of fasting in the old quarters and two days transit by boat to adapt them to new impressions. In a fast and prayer a double process takes place; not only will one lose interest in the old environment and the natural appetites, but the new consciousness goes on with great intensity, adjusting every faculty to the new focus. When we consider that this spiritual consciousness is the aim of our existence, its intensity, adjusting every fibre of our being toward that goal, becomes evident to us. In the new consciousness, we are empowered to receive new reaction to the old environment, which appears in a new light. This, of course, is realized to a fuller extent only when an individual sets himself on a long fast with much prayer and effort put forward while fasting.

"And He humbled thee, *and suffered thee to hunger,* and fed thee with manna, which thou knewest not, neither did thy fathers know; that He might *make thee know that man doth not live by bread only,* but by every word that proceedeth out of the mouth of the Lord doth man live." Deut. 8:3. This depicts in a wonderful manner how God wanted to change the environment of the children of Isreal so they could be changed and transformed

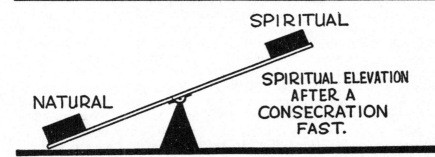

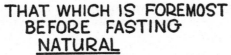

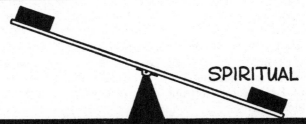

CHART No. XI. THE CHANGE IN ENVIRONMENT

Chart showing WHY ONE DOESN'T HAVE "FAITH AS A GRAIN OF MUSTARD SEED." THE CARNAL NATURE IS ELEVATED ABOVE THE SPIRITUAL. FASTING AND PRAYER LOOSEN THE NATURAL GRIP OF THE WORLD SO THAT THE POWER OF GOD AND FAITH BECOME MANIFESTED. Our body becoming neutralized is converted into a powerful spiritual conductor. After the flesh is arrested the Spirit charges.

ENVIRONMENT CHANGED TO SPIRITUAL GIFTS

Dear Brother Hall:

I can never tell you in words what the teaching of fasting and prayer, as set forth in your book, "Atomic Power with God," has meant to me I was earnestly seeking more on this subject, when this book fell into my hands. I simply devoured its great truth, backed by the word of God. Immediately I went on a consecration fast; God came on the scene and shortly I received gifts of healing.

I feel that you have the message of the hour, the one that will awaken the sleeping church, and cause men and women to become stirred to the realization that Jesus is coming soon. God is pouring out His gifts of the Spirit in these days. I attribute the success of my ministry to the message God gave you on fasting and prayer, that you so generously made many sacrifices to give to the body of Jesus Christ.

Your Sister in His service

Evangelist Thelma Nickel   405 South Wheeling Ave.   Tulsa 4, Oklahoma

*A song right out of Heaven: "I am the Lord That Healeth Thee." Received by Sister Nickel after fasting and praying. Order it from her at above address. Price 35c. Also see her book on divine healing, "Our Rainbow of Promise."   Price $1.00

from the habits and lusts of the old environment grip that the land of Egypt held over them. They were not in anyway adaptable to the new land of promise yet. The bondage of Egyptian environment was in their minds, body and soul. They still had lustful desires for the old things of sin, habit, program, and traditions of the world. Because they failed to accept the forced fast that was put upon them, by an all loving and wise Lord, they were required to break down this ENVIRONMENT the hard long way. By failing to fast and break down the bondage environment in a few days time and march right into the promised land, they were consequently compelled to march around in circles for forty years in order that the flesh could be broken and the old stubborn bound individuals died off, before taking the promised land.

We too can also miraculously change our Christian environment in ten days or longer of fasting that would otherwise require many long years of time and then it might be doubtful if as much progress could be made, the long way, outside of fasting and praying.

Our change in environment sometimes brings spiritual clairvoyance or visions. Moses, after his fasts, was enabled to actually see the presence of God Himself, with the result that the glory was reflected in his face ever afterwards. Often times the spirit of prophesy comes upon deep spiritual saints.

In Daniel 10:7: "And I Daniel alone saw the vision for the men that were with me saw not the vision.' Of course not, because only the prophet Daniel had fasted for twenty-one days with prayer, while his companions had not fasted.

Paul saw the angel sent to him on the thirteenth day of his fast. Paul saw the Lord. Acts 27:23. He was "in fastings often"; we may assume that fasting was one of the sources by which his vision was clarified.

Hermas, one of the church fathers, declares that the Lord appeared to him during a fast. Since the Lord is with us always, why should He not appear to those who will clear their eyes of doubt, bondage and unbelief with fasting and prayer? The fervent zeal of most of those who have declared they saw the Lord, could not have been the product of mere hallucinations. Many Christians after enforced fasts brought on by illness have claimed to have seen angels, their loved ones in glory, as well as the glories of heaven. The forced fast through illness, often drew them closer to God; new faith was acquired and they became healed.

St Thomas of Aquin, probably the greatest theologian of the Roman Catholic Church, fasted often, seeking revelation of the truth. This was finally given to him so gloriously that he refused to finish or add another word to the "Summa," a compendium of Roman Catholic theology which was to be his masterpiece. When entreated by friends to finish the work he refused, declaring all he had written hitherto to be but "rubbish" compared to what was revealed to him. If every devout Roman Catholic would seek the truth as earnestly as St. Thomas, with prayer and fasting, Romanism would soon be extinct. The glory of the Lord would soon be in the midst.

Most of the great revivals that have swept the land were born in fasting and prayer and could be traced back to that very thing. Some of the leading evangelists would prepare for the season of meetings ahead of time by a week or ten days of fasting and prayer. This accounted for the many healings and converts that they had.

Polycarp in A. D. 110 advises fasting to subdue the fleshly lusts and have better will power. Many old hermits and early church fathers used the fasting formula to obtain certain similar results.

FAITH PARALLELS FASTING

Faith cometh by hearing, and hearing by the Word of God. But in the Word of God Jesus has given us a more direct and specific pathway to the receiving of this FAITH. The disciples needed to fast in order to obtain faith to cast out certain demons. If unable to get victory over ordinary sicknesses and certain prayer accomplishments without fasting how much more should we fast, than the disciples? Surely this should spur us on toward fasting more than ever.

If faith is produced through Jesus' instructions on prayer and fasting, then there surely is a close relationship between fasting and faith. Shall we analyze both the subjects of FAITH and FASTING? Let us see how their relationship affects a person:

FAITH	FASTING
1. Faith ignores our sense faculties of sight, smell, taste, touch, and hearing.	1. Fasting wars against our members so that the senses, though keen in operation, will be subjected to the spiritual.
2. Faith ignores all feeling.	2. Our feelings change to a spiritual environment.
3. Faith works with the invisible.	3. Our miserable feeling is the subjugation of the flesh so that invisible spiritual power is manifested.
4. Faith is on a spiritual plane.	4. Fasting leads one into the Spirit.
5. "Faith worketh patience." James 1:3.	5. A major fast always gives one greater patience.
6. Faith is a substance.	6. Fasting brings one into contact with the substance of God.
7. Faith is the evidence of the unseen.	7. Fasting brings revelation evidence from God.
8. Faith ceases to be when the substance is made visible.	8. After the fast ends there is a major spiritual awakening.
9. Faith is anti-carnal.	9. Fasting is anti-carnal.
10. Faith is believing what is not seen by the natural.	10. Fasting takes one into an unseen spiritual realm, sometimes into visions.
11. Faith will bring one into the supernatural manifestation.	11. Fasting will undo the natural. It brings us into the supernatural.

12. Without faith it is impossible to please God.

13. Faith brings spiritual power.

14. Faith is the victory.

15. The natural man dislikes to believe in God.

16. Even Christians find it difficult to believe Christ for even their healings, which were bought for them.

17. Faith will "CAST DOWN OUR Reasoning." II Cor. 10:3-5

18. Faith pulls down the strongholds of the enemy. II Cor. 10:3-5

19. Faith operates on an invisible plane, bringing to light evil forces.

20. The more we exercise our faith the stronger we become in our Christian experience.

21. Faith will make a supernatural person out of an ordinary individual.

22. Faith works independent of the flesh.

23. Faith surprises the flesh by working unconventional to it.

24. Faith disregards the natural appetites and sometimes gives us supernatural appetites.

25. Faith can be a fruit of the Spirit and a gift. It is one of the greatest measures, to put into practice and develop in order to please God.

12. Fasting pleases the Lord.

13. Fasting produces the faith that leads to spiritual power and enters the Spirit realm.

14. Fasting moves God to victory for us.

15. The natural man dislikes to fast.

16. The children of the Bridegroom are urged to fast, yet it is so distasteful to them, seldom can one be found who has fasted ten consecutive days.

17. Fasting improves our natural memory, but seems unreasonable as to its value. Our reasoning is consequently mastered.

18. Fasting brings us into a great spiritual battle that ultimately brings great victory. See Daniel 10:2-14.

19. Satanic forces struggle against the fasting candidate, not desiring him to fast.

20. Fasting empowers a Christian to make great spiritual strides. To be our best we should be in fastings often.

21. Fasting neutralizes the flesh so that a person can become a powerful CONDUCTOR OF Spiritual power.

22. Fasting is disliked by the flesh.

23. Fasting is an anti-flesh measure giving the flesh it's greatest beating.

24. Fasting arrests the appetites so that they become dormant after three days.

25. Fasting and prayer can do more for a person and get that individual more closely to God than any other duties. It therefore honors and pleases our Jesus.

If you are not in the direct will of God, not as close to the Lord as you should be, or if you are called for service of the Master, YOU CAN BE YOUR BEST FOR GOD BY PRAYER AND FASTING. DON'T ARGUE ABOUT IT, TRY IT, "TASTE AND SEE," and you will be repaid a thousand times.

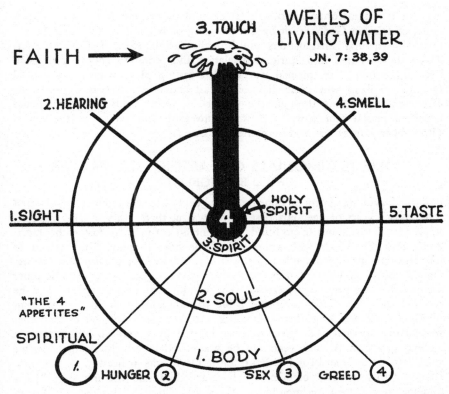

FAITH →

3. TOUCH

WELLS OF
LIVING WATER
JN. 7: 38,39

2. HEARING

4. SMELL

1. SIGHT

HOLY
SPIRIT

5. TASTE

4

3. SPIRIT

2. SOUL

"THE 4
APPETITES"

SPIRITUAL

1. BODY

1.

HUNGER ②

SEX ③

GREED ④

Chart No. XII. The SPIRITUAL MAN ANALYZED AND DIAGRAM-
ED AFTER FASTING AND PRAYING. NOTE THE BAPTISM OF THE
HOLY SPIRIT IN THE HEART OF MAN WHERE THE SOURCE OF
THE "WELLS OF LIVING WATER" SPRING. ALSO, HIS FIVE SENSE
FACULTIES ARE DIRECTED FROM THE SOURCE OF POWER AND
FAITH IN THE SPIRIT, by the Holy Spirit.

THIS REPRESENTS THE IDEAL MAN WITH ALL THE APPETITES,
all of the members, and the body, soul, and spirit completely yielded to the
Lord for service. This man will "LOVE HIS APPEARING," and will be
looking forward to the real change that will take place in him when the
"Trumpet sounds." He has an abundance of the oil of the Spirit.

Faith is not based upon sense-governed reason, nor upon things man can
see, unless they can see spiritual things. Faith deals with facts. The Holy
Spirit seeks to have dominion of our body, soul and spirit.

"Sense governed reason," being carnal, is a stronghold which we must
CAST aside if we are to remove unbelief and have faith to fulfill God's
great commission. On the battleground of our senses is the battle of unbelief.
"Sense knowledge" is faith's worst enemy because it will not give the Word
of God first place. In the fight for FAITH and the removal of unbelief,
FASTING will so completely and effectually take control of our sense-reason-

ing that it is transformed into a different kind of reasoning. A spiritual reasoning of faith in God's Spirit by the renewing of our minds. (Romans 12:1). Even our natural imaginations are brought down. (See II Cor. 10:3-5). These are converted into Spiritual revelation and power to believe with positive faith action. The spiritual warfare that fasting plays against our natural faculties, explains why some disliked to fast and others seek to minimize its effectiveness. Fasting through the power of Jesus, leads us where sense governed reason cannot walk. A walk into faith and power of the Spirit. (Remember our senses make up the old man).

SOME TESTIMONIALS OF FASTING AND PRAYER
CHILD EVANGELIST

Little David was born in Phoenix, Ariz, Sept. 20, 1934. He sang his first song at two years of age. His first prayer was at three years of age. At five, Little David was about to go blind. He went on a three day fast with prayer, going into the woods with some other little boys to pray. Satan talked to him and tried to discourage him the first day, but he kept praying and fasting. On the third day he went into the woods again and his prayer became more intense, the fast became prayer too.. The windows of heaven opened and he received the Holy Spirit after the Bible pattern and instantly he was completely healed and came home shouting. At the age of six he had another wonderful experience. At seven he was injured by a taxi-cab and healed in answer to prayer. At nine years old he was called to preach. At that age his spirit left the body and for five hours Little David was in heaven, a great light flashed across in front of him and he was called into the ministry. "Jesus told me to go, open my mouth and He would fill it. I also received knowledge of many things that are going to come to pass," stated Little David.

There is more to it than what appears on the surface. Let us go back before he was born. Little David's father, Brother Jack Walker, was not seeing the souls saved; he became heavily burdened, crying out to God almost night and day, and still he wasn't satisfied. Then he undertook a fast in almost ceaseless agony and prayer for lost men and women. He received, from the sombre, laden heavens above, a ray of hope, although he did not know what it was all about. This much he did know and that was God had answered his prayer. Victory was felt without a shadow of doubt. This fast and prayer lasted for fourteen days. Immediately at the conclusion of this fast, a soul was given to the parents and nine months later his son was born. This child evangelist was to do more than his father could ever do and was very definitely in answer to the most fervent prayers and FASTING.

Child and women preachers are last day signs of Bible prophecy being fulfilled. See Joel 2:28.

REVIVAL IN NORTH BATTLEFORD SASK., CANADA

The news of this revival has gone to many foreign countries and the present move is the topic of conversation around the world. It is a revival of spiritual power, Heavenly Choir singing, Healings, gifts of the Spirit, prophecy and a general spiritual downpouring etc.

Three buildings on the Airport at North Battleford, Sask., composed Sharon Orphanage and Schools at its beginning in the fall of 1947. About seventy students

RESULTS OF FASTING AND PRAYING

gathered to study the Word of God and fast and pray. After about three months the revival suddenly began in our classroom where the entire student body was gathered for devotional exercises. Day after day the Glory and power of God came among us. Great repentence, humbling, fasting and prayer prevailed in everyone. Some fasted several weeks, others went longer. One person fasted forty-days. Before this we were up against a wall so to speak, not being able to accomplish what we thought we ought to accomplish for the glory of God. We were almost in despair seeking and searching for truth. Brother Walter Fredericks sent us Brother Franklin Hall's book, "Atomic Power With God Thru Fasting and Prayer." We immediately began fasting with our praying. Previously we had not understood the possibility of long fasts. The revival would never have been possible without the restoration of this great truth through our good Brother Hall. A second great event in preparation of our hearts was the coming of Brother Wm. Branham to Canada with his ministry of healing. The presence of so great a gift from God made us to know that all the gifts were far beyond any conception we had previously held concerning them.

The revival still continues and the sovereign glory and power of God pervades the entire area round about. Words cannot describe the deluge of glory and power that was among us. There was no loud talking or laughing, everyone walked quietly, and bowed in awe before the mighty moving of the Spirit of God.

For more particulars subscribe for "The Sharon Rose" above address.

By Brother Earnest Hawtin

40-DAY FAST TRANSFORMS LIFE

BEFORE

AFTER

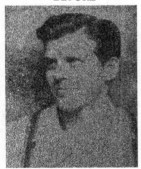

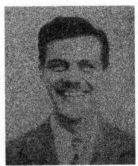

FORTY
DAY
FASTING

At the beginning of a 40-day fast. "I was proud, self confident, and self righteous."

I thought I had FAITH.

"On the fortieth day of my forty-day fast, without food. I learned more about God than all the rest of my life without Fasting."

J. A. Hida

J. A. Hida

Dear Doctor Hall:

Attached are pictures showing how I looked at the beginning and the end of my forty-day fast without food (water only). The first picture seems to express self-confidence and pride, while the second shows a confidence in God along with a more humble spirit.

I was drawn closer to the Lord by this fast than I could have been in years without fasting. The experiences were so wonderful that I want to go on another one just as soon as I get my weight back.

What I believe to be the most important truth in Dr. Halls's books on fasting, is that prayer must be fervent and much of it combined with fasting, if one expects to have the best results. When I learned this I began to really pray in earnest, and from that time on I have had no difficulty in praying. Fasting is also just as much for a person who cannot pray as for one who can (Psalm 35:13). It will help a person to be fervent in their prayers and receive answers to their hitherto unanswered prayers. Fasting makes Prayer effective and reawakens our faith (see James 5:16).

It is too bad that fearful and unbelieving folk do not konw what wonderful experiences they are missing in the prophet-length fast. If they knew, they would stop filling their stomachs right now and start tasting of divine glories! My fast was near Christmas time I had real anointing to give my testimony for Jesus and every day seemed like Christmas. I have had more boldness, wisdom, and spiritual power than ever before.

On the tenth day of the fast I had a heavy pull of prayer like as of travail. After that, prayer came easy. Weakness left me the seventeenth day. I felt wonderful, both spiritually and physically after that.

We need a revival in the land and I believe one is underway now and it will continue to grow and grow if we can get more and more saints loosened up enough to fast and pray to get their lamps trimmed and burning.

I was burdened for a spiritual re awakening in the "EAST," somehow I feel fasting will help.

Sincerely,
Jennings A. Hida
Box 385
Washington, D. C.

For more details of Brother Hida's 40-day fast, write to him.

FINANCIAL NEEDS MET—RECEIVED SPIRITUAL GIFTS AFTER FASTING TWENTY-ONE DAYS

Dear Brother Hall:

Fasting and prayer brought exceptional results in my life. I had some financial obligations to meet. The book, *"How to be a Successful Minister"*, of which I am the author, was ready for the press and there was but little funds for it to be published . . . Three hours after my fast was broken, Jesus sent in a large check for the publication of this book, from a stranger. A little later on in the week another check came in, making a total of $800.00. This was the necessary amount needed to get the book on the press.

After this publication, the Lord sent in many orders anointing the message in the volume, so that thousands have been blessed from the contents. (Many testimonial letters testify to this).

The Lord gave me much New Spiritual Strength in my life to pray for the sick. We sent out many anointed cloths all over the land and hundreds of testimonies poured in, telling how Jesus healed their bodies. I am thankful for the gifts of the Spirit that can come about through fasting and praying. There is no other book I have ever read outside the Bible that has done me so much good as "Atomic Power With God."

Yours in Christ,
Ted Fitch,
Council Bluffs, Iowa

WORLD-WIDE FASTING-PRAYER CRUSADE
————JANUARY 1946————

In 1946 a group of saints came together in San Diego, from various denominations, to hear the teaching of Jesus Christ's Gospel concerning prayer and fasting. Many of these Christians entered into consecration fasts. A real test was made as to the efficacy of fasting. Some of these fasts were from

Brother FITCH'S BOOKS ARE VERY VALUABLE AND HELPFUL
"How to be a Successful Minister" $1.25
"Our Afflictions, Their Cause and Prevention .... .75
These valuable books and others may be ordered from Brother Fitch at above address. Just write to him at Council Bluffs, Iowa.

twenty-one to more than sixty days in continuous duration without food. They were burdened to see the Lord move in a special spiritual way. These and many others wanted to see a world-wide revival for the salvation and healing of mankind and the restoration of the gifts of the Spirit.

The result of these scores of Christians fasting and praying was stupendous. Many miracles of healing were performed by the Holy Spirit in the Name of Jesus. Demons were cast out, lunatics healed, cancers disappeared, the blind saw, the crippled walk, stomach ulcers disappeared, palsy quieted, tuberculosis healed, asthma, bronchitis, the smoking and drinking habits were given up and many more sicknesses vanished. Scores of folk were baptized at the altars.

In this revival auditorium that the author was temporarily in charge of, we were privileged to see a thousand souls find Jesus that year. These converts were mostly service men from various parts of the nation. They also helped to carry the message into other areas.

A continuous chain of fasting and all night prayer meetings conducted by Sister Helen Hall, went on for many months. It was in the midst of these fasting prayer revivals that this volume was born. From thereon God burdened the author to launch a fasting and prayer crusade. This soon became world-wide in scope. Brother Dale and Barbara Hanson, who were with us while this book was under preparation also caught the vision to do their part. Soon many other ministers and spiritual saints of God also became burdened to encourage and teach prayer and fasting in a greater way. Folk began fasting in Los Angeles and Southern California and then it spread thru out the West and North into Canada. Then folk began fasting and praying across the nation. Soon this most powerful message had gone throughout the world. Men and women travailed in the most powerful prayer, the prayer prayed under the influence of a consecration fast. Such hunger and travail moved the hand of God and opened the windows of Heaven and God poured out His Spirit and Power in a mighty way.

Many calls, yes thousands of letters would pour in from all parts of the world asking for information on the deeper fastings. Truth that would take them deeper and deeper with the Lord and open up the doors so they could have more of the Holy Spirit and His gifts. Even before "Atomic Power With God," was off the press, orders had come in for approximately five thousand copies and requests for thousands of pieces of literature. There was a major financial problem, but our Lord supplied the need and members of the body of Jesus made it possible to print even millions of tracts on a subject most neglected and overlooked, yet at our very finger tips.

Thousands of wonderful testimonies would pour in from all over the world verifying the mighty power of fasting and prayer. They testified to God answering in their fastings like many testify to God answering prayers, only the fasting-prayer is more effectual.

The author launched fasting and prayer revivals throughout the nation. Auditoriums were filled with crowds varying from a thousand to fourteen thousand. These were non-sectarian for all churches. (See author's book, "The Fasting Prayer"). This started thousands of people to fasting and praying for a world-wide revival and this preceded, being a prelude to the major evangelistic healing campaigns that are stirring Christendom today where even thousands are converted in a single campaign.

Dark clouds of doubts and unbelief hovered over the church. The signs were not following believers as they should. Denominational barriers also prevented the full workings of the Spirit. Faith was without many works and was seemingly dead in many places. James 2:17: "Faith, if it hath not works is dead, being alone." Before there could be active faith in the body of Christ, to produce "signs following," (in a greater manner) the dark clouds of unbelief had to be penetrated and removed. According to Jesus' teachings in the seventeenth chapter of Matthew, prayer and fasting will remove UNBELIEF.

CONCLUSION

We have prophesied a number of places in our writings: "A great spiritual awakening is in the making. A mighty revival of power, signs, wonders and miracles are coming. The operations of the Holy Spirit will move with greater power when more folks catch the vision and go into prayers and fastings, as was done in days of old." Thousands of Christians have consequently gone into fasting from ten to forty days all over the world in behalf of a world-wide revival and more spiritual power.

Brother Wm. Branham in his healing meetings, led the way in proving to the world that Spiritual gifts could be exercised in a far greater manner than the average person had thought possible. Soon hundreds of other devout men and women who also received gifts of the Spirit were mightily used of God. Many times multitudes of sick folk having deafness, cancers, tuberculosis, ulcers, blindness, lameness, arthritis and scores of other diseases, many of which were incurable by man's power, were gloriously healed through FAITH in Christ's atonement.

Many of the gifts of the Spirit are being stirred up in Holy Spirit filled people. As men and women continue to fast and pray, more doubts and unbelief are being removed. A closer fellowship and harmony is also being restored among His members.

We feel we are only in the beginning of the greatest revival the world has ever seen and more miracles and operation of His Spirit will be manifested.

Praise the Lord; Jesus Christ is the same yesterday, today and forever. Let us all have signs following through fasting and prayer.

If you have not read the other volumes of this set, be sure to order and carefully read them. Many order extra books and help spread this truth among their friends. This is doing a missionary work for Jesus and you will be doing a blessing. *"Withhold not good from them to whom it is due, when it is in the power of thine hand to do it."* Proverbs 3:27. Pass the light you have received on to others. Knowledge brings responsibility.

If you will also mail in names and addresses of Christians, we will mail out free literature on this subject.

May Jesus bless you.

★

CPSIA information can be obtained
at www.ICGtesting.com
Printed in the USA
BVOW03s1751080617

486258BV00004B/203/P